EMILY SOUTHWOOD

PRUDE

LESSONS I LEARNED
WHEN MY FIANCÉ
FILMED PORN

SEAL PRESS

PRUDE
Lessons I Learned When My Fiancé Filmed Porn

Seal Press
Copyright © 2013 Emily Southwood
Published by
Seal Press
A Member of the Perseus Books Group
1700 Fourth Street
Berkeley, California
www.sealpress.com

Library of Congress Cataloging-in-Publication Data

Southwood, Emily, 1978-
Prude : lessons I learned when my fiancé filmed porn / Emily Southwood.
pages cm

ISBN 978-1-58005-498-0 (pbk.)
1. Southwood, Emily, 1978- 2. Pornography. 3. Women—Sexual behavior. 4. Sexual freedom. I. Title.
HQ471.S68 2013
306.7—dc23
2013023340

9 8 7 6 5 4 3 2 1

Cover design by Briar Levit
Interior design by Domini Dragoone
Printed in the United States of America
Distributed by Publishers Group West

FOR ROBBIE

CONTENTS

HAND JOB

It's one in the morning, and I'm sitting in my nightgown, scarfing single-serving microwavable lasagna. I've had a few gin and tonics; I've been out celebrating the end of grad school. Now I'm tipsy, ravenous, and contemplating how I'll pack up my disheveled apartment and vacate in three days. I'm shipping off to LA! For a boy! Or a man, which I guess is what I should call him at this rather adult juncture in life. I'm countable hours away from ending a two-year long-distance relationship, and—this just in—we're engaged! I look down at my floor-length, plaid, Laura Ingalls Wilder number, aware it's not a good look for a twenty-eight-year-old woman. Tonight is the last time I'll loaf in its cozy hideousness. Tomorrow it goes in the trash, along with most of my dismal surroundings. So long, three-hundred-square-foot spinster apartment! Adios, revolting, flower-curtained, mold-ridden communal bathroom that I share with an actual middle-aged divorcée! Ta ta, silverfish slinking through my cutlery drawer in this godforsaken, damp Vancouver climate. Some say it's paradise up here—the snowcapped mountains! The majestic freaking ocean! I say it rained thirty days in a row last month. Fuck the rain forest. I've disembarked from my last moist ride up to the university on the 99 B-line, with its vague smells of dog shit and packed lunches. California, here I come. My baby awaits me in the sunshine. I will sleep naked from now on; I'll wear vintage kimonos to fetch the morning paper on the electric-green lawn.

This will be my tenth move in my twenties. I've lived with a guy only once before. It didn't end well, actually. We were twenty-three, broke, and had a third roommate—a girlfriend of mine. Post-breakup, my ex refused to move out. I moved my bed into the living room. He stayed on for an extra month and routinely dumped Ritz crackers under my sheets.

I have a better feeling about this one. Being engaged lends a certain permanence to the whole thing. Who knew I could find that a comfort? Until recently, I hadn't thought of myself as the marrying kind. But life is full of unexpected little twists, like the phone call I'm about to receive from my fiancé, Robbie, telling me he's been offered a job filming on porn sets. I find the trilling portable under a marked-up draft of my thesis.

"I'm still on set, but I had an interesting day," my fiancé says. "I had a job offer."

"No way! For what?"

"Yeah, it's great. Kind of an interesting project though . . ."

"Interesting is good."

"It's as cinematographer for a reality TV show called *Webdreams*."

"Wetdreams?"

"No, *web* dreams. It's about porn stars."

"What?" I say. "What about porn stars?"

"Well, everything, I guess. I want to tell you about it because I have the interview first thing in the morning, but I have to keep working. Will you be up in two hours?"

"It's one in the morning. Will you accept the job if they make an offer?"

"I don't know. We'll talk about it. I forgot it was this late—this is a crazy shoot. Should I call you in the morning?"

"Call when you're done, I'll answer." I curtly click off the phone and place it on the coffee table. I stare at the benign plastic buttons for a moment, trying to compute what just went down. Did my fiancé tell me that he's taking a job filming *porn?* I think he might have. But maybe not? How *much* reality is there in reality TV porn? I have questions. What will this mean? Do I have a say in it? Why did he tell me about this at one in the morning, on set, I wonder? I start to feel anxious. The feeling is familiar. It's recognizable from two years of waiting up for calls from Robbie when I should have been able to just read a book and go to sleep. My foreboding feeling is also familiar because porn has always made me a touch uncomfortable . . . but I thought I was over that. I thought I'd been through my bona fide sexual liberation.

A few things to know about me in this moment: I've been with twelve guys and one girl; so I'm no Virgin Mary, but hardly Samantha Jones. More importantly, I don't think of myself as a prude. I wasn't chaste with Robbie. It was a warm June evening in 2004 when we locked eyes across a bar. I was bartending in a slip of an outfit; he was buying drinks and tipping well. I'd known him as an acquaintance for years but never thought of him that way until, *wham*, he was ripping my underwear off from under my miniskirt, the two of us mashed against a bathroom door. He smelled amazing—like April-fresh towels mixed with salty, summer skin. It was, by far, the most brazen affair I'd ever had. The attraction was tsunami-esque. We proceeded to hook up, late at night, every week or so, and thusly screwed our way around Montreal for half a year. We barely talked. I was tremendously pleased with this version of myself because I'd been mostly a serial monogamist. There I was, getting jiggy with no promises. It was my version of girl gone wild. Then he told me he couldn't keep seeing me if I didn't want to commit. He had *feelings*—shit. I dumped him promptly. However, double crap, it turned out I was rather attached too. Our breakup lasted one week.

Three years later, here I am—all in.

When it comes to my opinions of porn on this rainy, fateful night, as a fourth-wave feminist (or whatever tier I'm in) I've always assumed it's degrading. Assumed, because to be honest, I've never watched all that much of it. I was a teenager in the late nineties, back when Jenna Jameson was the height of hot, and the Internet was climaxing to billions of X-rated dollars, but I was totally oblivious. I was on my pink duvet getting off to a racy bit in a John Irving novel—a few images that incidentally served my masturbation needs for the better part of a decade.

Most porn I have seen has been with Robbie. He's been much more open about his taste for XXX than other guys I've dated. We've even watched a few videos together in an attempt to maintain my free-loving persona. My reaction has gone like this: a fluttering in my nether regions, followed by mucho critical analysis—*Does she really like that penis ramming down her throat like that? Hmmm? I've never cum from twenty minutes of jackhammering (let alone screamed with ecstasy the entire time). Are we still wearing Lee Press-ons, ladies? What's with the dudes in nothing but tube socks?* Nevertheless, I've made an effort to be accepting of Robbie's relationship with porn because I've made an effort to be accepting in general in this relationship. I've gone to the dark side with boyfriends before—probing and picking, searching for truths I didn't want to hear, only to have them confirmed. I've experienced what it's like to be in a never-ending tug-of-war, and I don't want that.

Not here. Not now. We're engaged.

If my twenties have taught me anything, it's that life is full of grey zones. I was once the kind of girl who used to feel annoyed when a guy opened doors for me and picked up the tab. I've come to appreciate such behavior, right along with the lipstick and heels I once eschewed. Besides, this relationship has been a reversal of many gender stereotypes. Namely, that Robbie talks about his feelings more than any man (or anyone) I've ever known. He doesn't do irony. The man can earnestly enjoy a Sarah McLachlan ballad. But he also likes to watch sports and porno. Now he'll be filming it. So what's the problem? Maybe there isn't one.

I think I need a cup of Sleepytime tea, or better yet, another drink. I pour myself some week-old white wine and run a bath. Reclining in nearly scalding water always makes me feel better. But my brain is busy with the news I've just learned. To boot, I'm feeling increasingly annoyed that Robbie decided to pop this grenade in the wee hours when he couldn't talk. Wouldn't I have been better equipped to deal with this over a cup of morning coffee? Am I really going to move to LA where my man films porn all day? Why does this proposition make me want to reconsider this whole commitment shebang? Am I secretly a right-wing conservative? How could I have anything in common with Sarah Palin? Maybe I'm simply way ahead of myself here, and *maybe* the show is a thoughtful study of contemporary culture. Perhaps I should call back and ask. The hot water is making me dizzy, so I towel off, return to the couch in my robe, and without thinking, dial.

"What's up?" he says. "I'm still working."

"I know, sorry. I have questions."

"I really can't talk."

"Then why did you call and tell me this in the middle of the night?"

"I'm sorry. I didn't think it was a big deal."

"Really? You don't think filming porn is a big deal?"

"I can't do this now."

"Fine." I hang up the phone and instantly regret it—both hanging up and calling. This is not the way to prove that I'm accepting and evolved, because, well, I'm not accepting and evolved right now. It's pouring rain and nearly two. I turn on the TV at a barely audible volume so my craggy downstairs neighbor won't get out his damn broom and start pounding on his ceiling. I'm restless. I'd go for a walk if there weren't a fucking monsoon. I'd pace the apartment if two steps in any direction wouldn't face-plant me into a wall. Just a few hours ago, life seemed on the up. Now I feel like a distinctly pathetic, and increasingly angry (mostly at myself), human being.

An hour later the phone rings on the coffee table, startling me out of my half-sleep.

"Hey," I say.

"You're still up?"

"Sort of."

"Why don't I call you in the morning?"

"No," I say, "I shouldn't have called back, but I wanted to talk." I sit up on the couch and wrap myself in a blanket to fetch some water. I drained the stale Sauvignon Blanc and I feel hungover—my head is fuzzy and aches.

"It's okay," he says. "I get it."

"You do?"

"Yeah, it's not just a normal job."

 "Are you taking it?"

"I want to talk to you about it before I make any decision. I'm not going to take it if you're not okay with it."

"You're not?" I exhale, feeling relief. I sit back on the couch and drink my water.

"Of course I won't. But we should really talk tomorrow; I'm tired."

"So you're going to be filming people schtupping?"

"Yeah, the producer said it's pretty graphic."

"Right."

"The show's for a major Canadian network, and they want a Canadian living in LA, so it could be a really good opportunity for me, for us."

"How's the pay?"

"Good, probably, but I'll find out everything tomorrow."

"I'm not exactly the world's biggest fan of porn."

"I know."

"I don't know how I'm supposed to feel about this."

"That's because it's weird—you're not alone. I guess they had someone else lined up who bailed at the last minute because his wife vetoed it."

"I wish you hadn't told me tonight."

"I'm sorry, I wasn't thinking. But it wouldn't really be any better tomorrow."

"What do *you* think about it? Are you cool with it?"

"Yeah, I'd be okay with it," he says. I pause.

"Of course. What guy is going to turn down shooting porn?" I say.

"I'm sure the porn factor will wear off pretty quick. It's more about the opportunity."

"Right."

"You don't believe me?"

"I guess. So if I'm not comfortable with this, I'm going to be blowing a huge opportunity for you."

"Don't think of it like that."

"How should I think of it?"

"I can't tell you that, sweetie."

We sit in silence for a moment. I hear his breath becoming heavier and sleepy. Some nights we fall asleep like this with hot phones to our ears, or at least he does, and I eventually hang up so that I, too, can drift off. My man has no such sleep difficulties.

"I want to be okay with it," I say.

"I know. I'll call you after I meet with the producer and director. I won't take it until we talk more, promise."

"Okay."

"I love you."

"Love you, too."

I hang up and sink back into the couch.

If I knew then what I know now, five years later, I would know that, as they say, things were going to get a whole lot worse before they got better. I would hand my former self a steamy cup of tea and say, "Oh, sweetie, this is just the tip." Pun wholeheartedly intended and relished in. I can make jokes like that now. While many women may not have had a problem with this scenario, I did at the time. Porn brought up extremely conflicting and nuanced reactions in me.

Some may know exactly what I mean when I say this, because they, too, have mixed feelings about XXX. Maybe you've suddenly become judgmental when stumbling upon an image with a caption like, pardon my French, "Big tit whore takes 3 black cocks" on your significant other's laptop. Then, perhaps, masturbated to it, felt shameful and gross, and subsequently pounded a large bag of Ruffles. No? Okay, that was probably just me; but see what I mean by conflicted? (This is, incidentally, the same exact, ambivalent response I have to the TV show *The Bachelor*.) Anyway, porn was both a turn-on and a turnoff. The turnoff part was harder to address and explain. Why? It's not that cool to be uncool with pornography these days or express opinions that can be synonymous with "ball-busting."

Personally, I've never wanted to be the prude girl, and I've gone to great lengths to avoid seeming that way. Only to inevitably wind up coming across as pretty damn uptight.

Since you're going to be getting to know me intimately, let me first delve into my sexual history in a little more detail. I guess I should start with how in 1992 I had a devastating crush on a boy named Justice. I was fourteen; he was fifteen. Our first "date" was in a park a few blocks from my suburban home, where I gave my paramour a semipublic hand job. He undid his button-fly Levi's for me to get things rolling. Then we lay on our sides and pressed into each other, exchanging warm, wet tongues. I'm right-handed and my right arm had fallen asleep under his head. So I went in with the left. It was a C– performance at best, and yet, thanks to teenage hormones, a few tugs later—voilà. Justice was not alone in his ecstasy. I had my first experience of what I would come to discover was my aptitude for the basically hands-free orgasm. I felt kind of racy, kind of grown-up.

Alone in my bedroom that night, I listened to Aerosmith's *Crazy* on repeat for three solid hours and incessantly wrote our names together in hearts. We hung out twice after that. He was my boyfriend, I figured. I thought a lot about what we would do for Valentine's Day. It was June.

Unfortunately, Justice didn't share the same level of deep, passionate feeling. He took off with a girl named Becky, who had a bit of a reputation, to follow the Grateful Dead. It was the nineties, not the seventies, but with a name like Justice he was bound to be nostalgic. I was heartbroken. I wished he had cared enough to wait for me to be ready to go all the way. Not until, like, marriage, but at least a few years. Oh well, I guess neither my bad lefty hand jobs nor my winsome personality were incentive enough for him to stick around.

Thanks to Justice, I learned that sex was collateral. Boys had to like you a lot or else they'd ditch you once they had what they wanted—be it a hand job in the park or your virginity. Our dad's speeches about "boys' intentions" were on point, after all. Armed with my new learning, I proceeded to cause numerous cases of blue balls among my teenage suitors. My ability to get off from a wee bit of dry-humping created quite the double standard.

By eighteen, I was ready to lose my virginity. For some reason, I treated it more like a business transaction than a starry night. One might infer that I had some control issues. I set my sights on a friend's older brother, Stephen, who was responsible and kind—a prudent investment my accountant dad approved of. On the appointed night, we did it in my bedroom, with my parents snoring down the hall. Stephen was a complete gentleman. He congenially wrapped the condom in a tissue, kissed me goodbye, and snuck out without a sound. When he called the next day to check in, I dumped him. The gist of it was this: he liked me too much, like, bordering on love. Don't ask me why this always had a reverse effect on me—love, presumably, being something you want boyfriends to feel about you. Not me! Not if they beat me to it. If anyone liked me more than I liked them at the time, it just completely made me want to dry-heave.

In university, I met my first love (and second lover). I was completely nuts about him from the second I spotted his goatee in African Literature class. The clear approach was to follow him on the Montreal Metro. My stalking paid off by midterms when I bought a pack of cigarettes, even though I didn't really smoke, and bummed a light from him outside the

DeMaisonneuve exit. (I knew he was a light smoker because of my sleuth detective work.) Then, in an extremely loud voice, I said: "Hi! My name is Emily!!!" He looked at me funny, both because I was addressing him like Helen Keller and because I was dressed like Ani DiFranco. Nevertheless, he introduced himself as Sam.

We stayed together for four years, which, at that age, is the equivalent of a twenty-year marriage. In this relationship, I grew more sexually comfortable, confident, and expressive; however, I knew I needed a few more spins around the block before any possibility of settling down. I could not be a worldly woman, having slept with only two people. Breaking up was long and arduous, and involved several sessions of dust-busting cracker crumbs from my sheets. Eventually, I cut the cord in pursuit of casual sex and reclaimed the bedroom.

I proceeded to learn a thing or two about regular STD tests, tugging on your dress at dawn, and keeping spare skivvies in your purse. In truth, I never did the single thing for long. Before I knew it, I was getting to know so-and-so's mom during weekends on the hippie farm where he grew up, then abruptly dumping him with zero explanation after six months. On the one hand, my ineptitude for small talk, inability to mask my emotions, and general wariness of strangers made me ill-suited for casual affairs. On the other hand, my "Don't love me first" dogma made me a tad difficult to deal with in serious relationships.

Obviously, I was a real riot to date.

At twenty-six, I was wholeheartedly trying to remain unattached when I met Robbie. Remember? June night, miniskirt, up against the bathroom door? Warning: this is not a recommended method for landing the man of your dreams—or so says those snobs who wrote *The Rules* and that Neanderthal who published *He's Just Not That Into You*. Our sexual dynamic was the most open I'd ever experienced. Robbie knew what he liked and wasn't shy about sharing it; he inspired the same candor in me. On my first sleepover at his apartment, he unabashedly donned a t-shirt with nothing else and hopped into bed. "What? My shoulders get cold at night," he said. As everybody knows, a man in just a t-shirt isn't hot. Basically, the man has no shame.

When the topic of pornography came up one night over pillow talk, he was equally blunt. At least compared to the sensitive-new-age-guys I'd dated before who'd either genuinely disliked porn or, more likely, sugarcoated their XXX consumption. These men were a product of single mothers and the PC nineties. If they'd watched porn, they'd kept it on the down-low, lest they feel judged by a woman in Birkenstocks. (Apparently some of us girls had a bit of a death stare.) I'd always backed up my discomfort around porn with feminist arguments. I was resolute that no woman would enter that profession by choice. I certainly wouldn't suggest it to my offspring, alongside professions like doctor or journalist. I also remained oblivious to the fact that porn was rapidly becoming available to every tween with WiFi, and never explored it for myself. So when Robbie asked me my opinions of porn, I held my tongue. I liked my increasingly liberated sexual self. Maybe I had something to learn from this openly porn-consuming guy? One thing was for sure—I didn't want to be an uptight, nut-squeezing bitch.

He suggested we watch some together one night and whipped out his laptop. Before I knew it, I was witnessing a blonde mash her massive tits facedown on a washing machine and take it up the ass. Then she turned, planted her bare knees on the concrete and let him ejaculate in her mouth. *Huh, so that's what I've been missing.* Don't get me wrong, I was turned on by the purely physical aspect of seeing people have sex, but the subservience of the girl in the scene made me uncomfortable. *Is this what guys expect? No way she was loving that, was she?* Robbie and I had sex that night (albeit not in the demonstrated manner), and I avoided talking about my feelings as I'd avoided math class in high school.

After a year of dating, Robbie and I both moved away to attend graduate school in different cities—he in LA and I in Vancouver. We decided to stay together. In between our tearful goodbyes and heartfelt promises, Robbie made another grand gesture of commitment—giving me his porn collection via memory stick. "We can watch it together," he said. By this point, I thought we were hugely evolved in our sexual communication. Who was this guru-slash-man who had no qualms sharing everything with me? "He's so open about sex, he even shares his porn!" I bragged to my friend Kate. I figured we must have been reaching relationship enlightenment. In truth, we never really wound up watching it much, and when we did, I still had mixed reactions—something could turn me on but then strike me as degrading in an instant, feelings I still never addressed with him.

Robbie called me back the next day to say he'd been offered the job and that the decision was ours to make. If I felt strongly about him refusing it, he would happily turn it down and not look back. But we had another big factor to consider: our enormous student debt. *I'm talking six figures.* Not to mention, my refusal to be a pushy woman meant I wasn't about to tell him he couldn't do something. So I lied, just as I had when watching porn with him. I didn't want him to do it, so naturally I said, "Take the job!" I ignored my deeper feelings because I was more concerned with the impression I was making. *Talk about commitment to not being bossy.*

The next eight months found me waiting for my fiancé to come home from the gang bang, while wishing to the good lord (a.k.a., my vague belief in karma, astrology, and "the universe") that I could travel back in time and tell Robbie not to accept the position. Little did I know, however, that this struggle would ultimately make our relationship stronger and change many of my opinions on pornography. My experience also prompted me to undergo an exploration of our cultural relationship with smut. *Hint, hint*—it's pretty conflicted. Some point to porn's harmful influence, while others advocate its value—or, as in Utah, many consume and condemn it all at the same time.

Here's a gem about influence: Apparently, college-aged girls these days are getting their first glimpses of smut on the Internet at eleven (thanks, *New York Magazine*, for that insightful bit!). There's more! These young women also confirmed that porn influences their boyfriends' expectations—and how *couldn't* it, when they're learning about sex from a couple of hot, bi-curious, waxed-bare blondes? Talk about raising the bar. In a tale as old as time—only with new media—the girls snapping topless iPhone shots and texting them to the boys are labeled sluts by the other girls and revered by the guys, if for a minute. While some things never change, there's a yawning chasm between what happens online and what happens with the girl next door, who isn't always a MILF in a cheerleading uniform. *And by MILF, of course, I mean a nineteen-year-old whose surgically repositioned nipples have never seen a teething baby.*

I'm not the only one who sometimes feels like a prude in the face of pornography these days. The subject of XXX puts many people on edge; I used to be one of them. Sex alone is often an awkward discussion topic, which sensibly we'd sometimes rather avoid. When's the last time you brought it up with your significant other in conversation? Honestly. Have you talked to your kids about porn? Are these discussions we *should* have? All I know is, I'm better off because I had them. My relationship is too. But heaven knows I would have dodged more chats about squirting if they hadn't come up in response to "Hi, honey, how was your day?" I *never* thought the answer would be "Super soaked." Sorry if that's TMI. I've definitely lost some perspective on what's appropriate dinner conversation.

Actually, I beg forgiveness in advance if I'm occasionally crass from here on out. I've discovered that YouPorn categories (YouPorn .com, for anyone who doesn't know, as I once didn't, is a free porn website) can be pretty good metaphors for life. Suffice it to say, if the next eight months were a TV show, every second word would be bleeped. With my fiancé filming behind-the-scenes of *Gang Bangs of New York*, conversations that may not have occurred over fifty years of marriage, if at all, occurred in weeks.

I was reluctant and even resentful to find myself contemplating the role of pornography in my relationship while I designed wedding invitations. (There isn't a how-to on porn in *Brides* magazine, ladies. I checked.) The experience revealed cracks in our relationship's foundation. I discovered fears I didn't know were there, and reservations I'm ultimately grateful I confronted. And of course, along the way, I thought and learned a heck of a lot more about porn than I ever wanted to. Prude? You be the judge.

CHAPTER 1

SQUIRTING

I'm in Los Angeles for Robbie's film school graduation. It's supposed to be my official move-in with my husband-to-be, but the Department of Homeland Security has negated our plans. They have a way of doing that sort of thing. It seems I'll have to return to Canada to finalize some paperwork. In the meantime, Robbie's whole family—both sets of parents, two siblings, and one sister-in-law—are all here. I'm technically still borderline family. A wife, one legal signature removed.

It's a foggy, grey afternoon in June—the one month out of the year that you *can't* count on sunshine in LA. Robbie and I are hanging out in his room before meeting his mom and stepdad for dinner. Robbie's convinced me that it's a good idea to watch an episode of *Webdreams*, season one. It makes sense to see what he's actually going to be filming rather than imagine it, is the thinking.

It's been about a week since he said yes to the job offer—"Yes, I will film porn stars in all manner of crude encounters. No, I won't pop

a boner." I'm still adjusting. And by adjusting, I mean stifling the discomfort that emerges every time the new job is mentioned. I can't even
think about what this anxiety is, why it exists; all I can do is stuff it down.
Swallow hard. I'd prefer not to think or talk about it. But the consensus
so far is that people think a job filming porn stars is something to talk
about. Basically, the topic comes up a lot. And each time, I perfect my
poker face: a look of bemused disinterest. A look, come to think of it,
perfected by porn stars.

So it is that Robbie and I are lying next to each other—all lanky, six-
feet-two inches of him alongside the wee five-feet-two of me. We watch
a hot brunette get busy with a busty blonde on his fifteen-inch laptop.
There's a bright pink dildo involved. The blonde reclines on a bed with her
double D's splayed apart—as much as silicon splays, that is—and moans.
They've been at it for a while (about twelve decades, in my estimation)
and the blonde is having trouble cumming, or rather *squirting*—which
I've just learned is an unfortunate colloquialism that evokes mustard bottles but actually means "female ejaculation."

Alternatively, Robbie tells me, it's sometimes called *gushing*—a
word that like *moist* and *panties* also makes me want to wretch bile. The
brunette cheers the blonde on in a sexy-meets-soccer-coach voice: "Yeah,
that's it! Cum for me, baby!!" And a very long two minutes later, she does,
like a stream emerging from a wide-mouthed cherub on a Venetian fountain, or a fire hose turned on a blazing building, or the gas pumps spray-
ing in *Zoolander*. You get the point. I shift uncomfortably, uncrossing
and recrossing my legs.

"No way that's real," I state unequivocally, glancing over at Robbie
to gauge his level of interest. His blue-grey eyes stare straight ahead. The
deep crow's feet that belie his twenty-seven years of age are fixed in a
forced, neutral expression.

"I've heard it is . . ." he says.

"Nah, she has a water balloon up there. See, this is what I mean about my suspension of disbelief, it always kills the mood for me."

"Maybe watching this wasn't the best idea." He hits Pause on the show, which is now following another set of characters—a woman and her husband, who stars in gay porn. But forget that for a minute, I still have my mind on the dog-and-pony show I've just seen performed. How have I managed to live nearly thirty years of my life and never hear of this? And why, again, is it coming up (or, *yikes*, squirting out!) now?

Just yesterday we sat on the lawn at Robbie's film school and listened to David Lynch and Sean Connery proffer up wisdom to the graduating class of aspiring filmmakers. They didn't mention that the bang bus was about to arrive with gainful employment. No, Sean Connery wore a kilt in the pomp and circumstance (much to the titillation of many a proud mother). He spoke of bright futures. And to be fair, landing a job filming a network-level reality TV show right out of the gates is no small thing. Even if it is a job that requires Robbie to trail porn stars in their daily lives—noshing low-cal lunches, hoofing it down to the tanning salon, and yes, filming all number of sex acts. And so here we are, discussing whether or not *squirting*—curse the gerund—is real. (Eventually I'll realize that it is sort of like debating whether Pamela Anderson has had a boob job. Anyway, live and learn.)

"So, you've obviously seen this before," I say, with the same not so subtly suspicious tone Oprah used when she interviewed Jenna Jameson.

"Yeah," he says.

"Lots of it?" I push, and quickly regret my Inquisition-style approach.

"Nah."

I fill in the silence, softening my tone to try to sound more curious and interested instead of judgmental: "So . . . you think it's sexy?"

"Um," he says, "I guess having a visual of a girl's orgasm is pretty hot."

"Right, I can sort of see that," I say, wondering why every time I try to sound open and accepting it comes out like I'd been sucking back helium. "Because you guys usually just have moans and facial expressions to go on."

"Right."

"And so getting splashed in the face with a bucket of pee is rewarding, in that sense." There, I said it. I couldn't help myself.

"It's not pee!"

"Uh huh, so *you* say."

"It's really not pee."

"Right, prove it then!" I mean to say this playfully, but it comes out sounding defensive. I then realize he'll actually have plenty of opportunities to provide evidence.

"Yeah, fine, I guess we'll see," he says, sounding faraway. He's checked out of this debate. As usual, he's forever attempting to keep the peace, which right now means aborting this heated topic. "We should get ready," he says. "I need to trim my beard." He reaches one hand to his face, juts his chin out, and scratches his brownish red scruff. Robbie's mom hates his beard long, but I think it's sexy. He's currently wearing it much longer than the short hair on his head, which he shaves to blend in with his bald spot. He's handsome bald—no Donald Trump dos here, thank God.

We have to be at the restaurant for dinner in half an hour. *Oh joy of joys,* straight from this conversation to chitchat with my soon-to-be in-laws. He leans over and briskly kisses me, punctuating the fact that we're moving on. I still kind of want to pry further. He would no doubt prefer to never revisit this Hallmark moment, unless it leads to actual sex rather than an awkward discussion about it.

I hop up from the bed and walk over to my suitcase to figure out something to wear. I'm terrible at packing and always wind up with too many sweaters in the tropics and too many tank tops for a ski trip. Predictably, my various sundresses don't fit the grey, chilly weather. I throw on a floral number and strappy sandals. Christ, I might as well be wearing a lei and slurping a mai tai.

"I'm going to miss you," Robbie says, still reclining on the bed, his eyes closed. His long, hairy legs extend from navy cargo shorts to black athletic-socked feet crossed at the ankles. His hands overlap across his stomach. He looks closed off, defeated. I feel bad. This didn't go the way he'd hoped.

"Am I going to dinner with your parents alone?" I joke. "That wasn't made clear to me." I know he's referring to our last stint of long distance while I file my visa, but I want to lighten things.

"Yeah, I'm going to stay here and watch these girls."

"Ha. Funny." I plop back on the bed and snuggle next to him. "You know, we're pretty close now."

We are both beyond done with the long-distance dynamic—ready to live in the same place, no more plane rides and constant goodbyes, hopefully less drama. And lucky for Robbie, no more B-grade phone-sex acting. I take full responsibility for my sexy telephonic failures. I gave it many, many a college try, don't get me wrong. But Robbie is, shall we say, more descriptive in the phone-sex department, while I would be fired from *Live Nude Operators* in two-point-five seconds flat for my unconvincing heavy breathing and Meg Ryan moans. And yet, for some reason, the poor man still wants to marry me. I must be much better in person; at least that's what I'm telling myself.

All in all, I can't believe I'm getting hitched. Believe me, I'm not the kind of girl who grew up daydreaming about her wedding day, dress and all. It was just never my fantasy, but I had other romantic delusions—a stable full of horses, a crackling fire, and a library full of books. I'd seriously debated the institution of marriage, particularly the idea of being someone's *wife*. It always smacked of sacrifice, housework, screaming children. That is, until Robbie proposed unexpectedly, without a ring, and I suddenly became the giddy star of every romantic comedy, bursting into tears with an emphatic yes. How the mighty crumble. So much for *The Feminine Mystique* . . .

"I can't wait to be here for real," I say, looking around. This will be my apartment too, and sprawling LA will be my home. But for the moment, we have to go. "What are you going to wear?" I ask. A mai tai is sounding better by the minute.

"A jacket probably," he says, the laptop still balanced on his thighs. "Roger will." Robbie's stepdad, an MBA professor in his seventies, is the kind of guy who wears a suit to go bird-watching.

"Okay, then!" I say, getting up from the bed. "Watch and be amazed . . ." I grab a shirt, tie, and jacket from his closet and toss them at my husband-to-be, a wifely gesture of sorts. "Time to put the porn away, dear. You don't want blue balls at the table with your parents." My attempt at levity is lost on Robbie, and he sighs as he shuts the computer.

As we sit at the restaurant with Robbie's mom, Lynn, and stepfather, Roger, my mind leaps between what Robbie will be filming and what to order. Mussels à la Marinière? Maybe not. We are sitting outside, so Robbie has lent me his jacket. Now I look like Ellen DeGeneres in Cancún. As usual, Lynn is dressed impeccably. Tonight she wears a grey silk blouse, plentiful silver arm bangles, and a coral pashmina draped across her shoulders. I try to listen to her story about their upcoming trip to Africa. My mother-in-law-to-be is explaining her travel itinerary in rigorous detail. I make a mental note to ask my best friend Kate her thoughts on this squirting phenomenon—*it's pee, has to be, right?* I hope nobody will expect me to remember any of these damn Safari details later. We haven't told them we're engaged yet. Robbie wants to do the traditional thing and ask for my hand in marriage (even though he already asked me first). We won't see my dad in person until August, so we've decided not to tell anyone about our engagement until then. It's an exciting secret. Currently trumped by the instant replay button malfunctioning in my head.

"And then we finish the tour with a trip to the vineyards around Cape Town!" Lynn says, wide-eyed.

"That sounds amazing!" I say, possibly a little too loud and vigorously, since Robbie gives me a sideways look.

"It'll be the trip of a lifetime, we hope!"

"Cheers to that," Robbie says. We all smile at one another and clink glasses. I take a long gulp of Pinot Grigio.

"And I guess we should say cheers to your new job, sweetie," Lynn says, her tone one of a mom trying to pretend it's not incredibly awkward to be toasting her baby boy for filming women having sex for a living.

"Yes, I guess we should, Mom," Robbie laughs.

All I can think is, *How weird.* But we've come to expect these tentative responses from our parents.

"I know it's not exactly a job you'll brag to your book club friends about," he says, teasing her to ease their mutual discomfort. He watches for her reaction with one eye. She gives a forced smile and intently spoons her potato-leek soup.

"Our only reservations, sonny," Roger interjects authoritatively, sitting straight-backed in a navy jacket and a well-matched tie, "are whether

having this on your resumé could have a negative impact on future jobs."
He stops and looks at me. "As well as that you *and* Emily feel comfortable
with this. I can imagine some women might find it intimidating to have
their boyfriend working with women who . . ." he pauses, clearly searching
for a word and vaguely gesturing to his chest region, ". . . you know," He
halts again, clearing his throat gruffly, and then quickly ejects the words:
"The type of physically endowed women that Robbie will be filming."

The three of them turn and look at me. I feel my cheeks ignite. At
the best of times, a table of people staring at me is enough to make me
blush. But a table of people questioning whether I and my A cups, not
to mention my love handles and cellulite, are intimidated by svelte porn
stars? That's just next level. It doesn't help that I resemble a lesbian on a
Carnival cruise. With nowhere to run, I choose the old fight response.

"Not me!" I say, all blasé confidence. "We've discussed it at length
and we're totally on the same page, right, luv?"

"Em has been amazing," Robbie concurs. He looks at me lovingly
and squeezes my knee under the table. "Besides, I think I'm the one who
might feel inferior." His joke gets a laugh, which thankfully takes the
attention off me. I instantly relax. He's good like that. Then we all turn to
our meals and change the subject to the gloomy June weather.

All in all, my new M.O. really seems to work wonders: *When in
doubt, lie.*

On my way home to Vancouver, I decide to kill time at LAX with a
call to Kate. I wander around the duty-free shop and begin my inquisition.

"*Is squirting for real?*" I hiss into the phone, as I pretend to browse
the lipsticks. "I just watched it yesterday in some, um, porn video, and
I'm not convinced."

"I'm not sure," she says. "I've heard about it but never experienced it."

"There's just *so* much liquid flying out, you know?" A woman looks at me sideways, and I make a beeline for the perfume. "*It's like Mount fucking Vesuvius!* I'm in duty-free, by the way, my flight's in a few minutes."

"I don't think that can be real. But on the other hand, I'm not sure it's the kind of thing you go around advertising either, you know? Why are we inquiring about this today?"

"The porn show, of course."

"Ah yes, when does that start?" she asks. "How are you feeling about it?"

"Fine, no biggie," I say. "It starts in a few days. What are you up to?"

"Okay then, we're leaving it at that?" she pauses, giving me a moment to divulge further, but I don't and she drops it. "I'm waiting for someone to come fix my garage door because I backed into it," she says.

"That's clever. Did it require a trip to emergency?"

"Very funny," Kate says. She is my close confidante for many reasons, but one of them is that she makes me seem extra-coordinated. One time she was standing on her bed to check out a miniskirt in the dresser mirror and gashed her head open on a ceiling fan. She'd purchased the skirt to make herself feel better about spending Valentine's Day alone. The cut required eight stitches. Despite being uncannily uncoordinated on the ground, Kate's a riding coach by way of profession. Go figure.

"You should really stop drinking and driving; it's unbecoming over thirty, like tube tops," I say.

"Sadly, I was sober. I'm on a cleanse, and I'm late. I need to get to the stables."

We hang up and I make my way to the gate after buying an over-priced iced coffee and some inane celebrity gossip rag to pass the time. I flip by "Stars! They're Just Like Us" without even registering how ridiculous the photos are of celebrities brandishing ice cream cones and frolicking with their kids on slides. Nope, I'm too busy wondering if any of these "stars like us" have mastered this *so-called* squirting.

A few nights later, Robbie and I are back in our respective cities catching up on the phone at the end of the day. I've been running around Vancouver dealing with bureaucratic nonsense. He's getting ready to start shooting the show the next day. We're both lounging on our beds, exhausted. I've just taken a bath and I'm in my robe, sporting a towel around my head.

"Maybe we should watch something sexy?" I suggest.

Since the squirting episode, I've been thinking that maybe a little more exposure to pornography would do me some good. We've watched it together before, after all, and it hasn't been all bad, truly. Besides, I want to show Robbie that I don't always have to be a judgmental and sarcastic psycho. I can be fun! It doesn't take a genius to recognize that my bad reactions probably discourage him from wanting to share his thoughts and feelings about porn with me. The pattern of this behavior is inevitable: he'll shut down; I'll feel left out. And I hate feeling excluded. I'm the baby of my family. I've self-psychoanalyzed that this feeling is part of my problem with pornography—it feels like a world just for men. A boys-only club; Virginia Woolf taught me to be wary of those. But I've come up with a solution. We'll watch more porn together! It will be a bonding exercise. I think I read about it once in a "How to Spice Up Your Sex Life" article in *Marie Claire*.

"Okay," he says. "Are you sure?" He sounds skeptical. "What do you want to watch?"

"I don't know, what are you into these days?" I say tentatively.

"Don't you want to pick?"

"I don't know where to start, really. It's your choice."

"Okay. If you're sure. Go to YouPorn.com and search: C-Y-T-H-E-R-E-A."

I type it in and several video clips pop up. I click on one and there she is. She's cute—a petite brunette with small boobs, not your traditional porn star, minus the copious iridescent eye shadow and weird bustier. She looks kind of like, well, me. Okay, me minus twenty pounds with injected lips, sporting '90s lip liner.

"I kind of like her look," I say.

"Me too!" my man replies, clearly encouraged by my reaction. "She's hot. I found her on YouPorn about a month ago and I like a lot of her stuff."

"So you watch her a lot?" I instantly regret my question, but the words have flown the coop.

"Um, yeah, I guess recently I have."

I ignore the feeling of jealousy that ignites when I think about all of the quality time he's spent with Cytherea. I'm determined to remain open-minded and not discourage him from sharing with me. We choose a video and press Play. Cytherea lies on a black-velvet throw blanket, fingering herself and making a face like she just bit into a lemon, then licking and biting like she wants to do it again—emotions I've seen more effectively conveyed in a high school drama class. A man, presumably Eastern European, enters the scene wearing nothing but combat boots and proceeds to head straight for her with his enormous, erect penis. Cytherea takes his supersized member into what I assume is her tiny vagina by the way she screams at the top of her lungs. Vladimir pounds away as if it's his job, which it is, and then abruptly retreats from the frame. Suddenly it becomes quite clear why—our gal pal Cytherea has a special talent.

"Good lord!" I yell, as the camera lens appears to have gone through a car wash. "That was quite the screen shot."

"Are you into it?" he asks. I don't quite know how to answer the question. Frankly, I'm not that into it, but the more pressing problem is that now all I can think about is how last week Robbie said that squirting wasn't a particular interest of his. But if he "likes a lot of her stuff," that sentiment doesn't exactly add up.

"I'm confused," I say. "I thought you said you weren't really into this."

"When did I say that?"

"When I was in LA and we were watching *Webdreams*."

"I did?"

"But the truth is, you really watch it all the time?"

"Sorry, I guess that was a bit of an omission . . ."

"I'm not sure I'm really in the mood anymore," I say. "Maybe we should talk tomorrow."

"Hey, don't go there," he says, but I'm already childishly hanging up. I look down at the phone and at the rather pathetic midcoitus scene I find myself in—vibrator in hand, porn paused on the screen, one boob hanging out of my bathrobe. It would be pretty funny to me if I weren't livid. I guess our attempt at show-and-tell didn't have the desired effect. I put my parts back in my bathrobe and walk to the living room. The phone rings.

"You really have to stop hanging up on me."

"How exactly are we supposed to be building trust when you're not being honest!"

"I guess I was afraid of what you'd think," he says. "You seemed really uncomfortable when we watched that episode in LA."

"I did?" *Apparently I'm not quite as stealthy as I like to think.* I can understand why he doesn't want his tastes judged, especially something clearly out of my norm. In my more rational mind, I can even appreciate why he's wary of my reactions. I am acting a wee bit like a lunatic. And yet, *grrrr.*

"I'm trying to work on my shit, and I feel like you're not meeting me halfway," I say.

"I get it, I'm sorry."

"Now I get to think about you heading off to shoot Jenna freaking Jameson tomorrow. I love my life."

"I'm not filming Jenna."

"Whatever, I know. It was just an expression."

"I don't want to get off the phone angry," he says. "Not tonight."

"What do you suggest? A squirter orgy?"

"No," he says, sounding like a kicked puppy. "I love you."

"Me and *Cytherea.*" I follow up my five-year-old retort with "I love you too."

We hang up and I make a cup of tea to bring to bed. An Ambien sounds better but my mom isn't around to steal one from. It's puking rain outside, of course. I lie in bed watching headlights cross my ceiling and thinking someone should write more country love songs about this sort of thing—porn ballads. *My baby told me lies, I had to tell him goodbye, now he's dreaming of getting soaked, I'm alone, watching the rain, feeling choked.* Maybe I just need to let go of the details and laugh at it all. Am I really threatened by Cytherea? Do I really feel inferior because I can't squirt? More importantly, is squirting even real? I decide to replay the scene for investigative purposes. By the fourth replay, I am no closer to determining whether Cytherea has some sort of magician's water bag up her vagina. If she does, I have no idea how she fits both it *and* Vladimir up there at the same time. By viewing number five I'm turned on, despite myself. I decide to tire myself out with some angry masturbation. Five orgasms later, I've discovered that it's entirely possible to hate-fuck yourself, all the while mentally reapplying someone's eye makeup.

The next day I awake to one distinct thought—my fiancé will be filming folks schtupping. I make coffee, throw on a muumuu and clashing sweater, surf headlines on the 'net, and still my brain prattles on—Robbie is filming people—a.k.a., hot chicks. I don't want to think about this. I don't want to revisit our fight. But my thoughts persist obsessively. Distraction is in order. I pack, do some edits on my creative nonfiction thesis, which is about my generation's delayed trudge toward adulthood, then call my mom to say that everything is going swimmingly! No luck. Mom's AWOL, probably chilling with her yoga pals.

Due to an overconsumption of bridal magazines, I've decided I have to lose my love handles before walking down the aisle. With that helpful diversion in mind, I drag myself down to "Total Body Conditioning" at the local community center. Our instructor's name is Shelly; she wears a headset and Spandex. Much to our delight, Shelly blares B-list pop songs and we follow along while she hops around like it's 1983. Shelly doesn't seem to give a shit what people think. I bet she can really let loose in bed.

Because of my British heritage (or that's what I blame it on, anyway) I'm extremely unattractive when I exercise. I sweat copiously, turn red, puff up—there's nothing ladylike about it, and for years it's been my vain reason for avoiding group sports. Thus, unsurprisingly, I'm not very good at athletics. Flailing around like a drunk blind person to Shelly's instructions with only middle-aged ladies from my neighborhood as witnesses, I really start grooving and begin to feel much better. This is what I need: to let go, focus on other things, like burning some calories doing squats to old Mariah Carey. *Except that the other jiggling asses in the room remind me of you know what.*

By the time I bike home I feel like Gwyneth Paltrow, when in fact I more closely resemble Ricky Gervais. Nevertheless, I haven't thought about what Robbie is zooming in on (like silicone and shaved cooch) for about twenty minutes, so things are looking up. I shower and decide to celebrate with an evening glass of wine. It is six, after all, and I figure I'll hear from Rob in about an hour, after the shoot is done. Wine will help the passage of sixty minutes. I put on some tunes and fix myself a meal—salad in honor of sticking with the program. Then I plunk down in front of the TV to eat.

Two hours of reruns and three-quarters of a bottle of wine later, there is still no word from Robbie. Tipsy, I decide I can't sit at home waiting for the post-porn phone call any longer. I don't have a cell phone, as I've been a poor student scrimping to save. But getting drunk at home while your fiancé films porn is too depressing, so I decide to go out and forgo waiting. I call some friends and we meet at a crappy bar on Broadway. Zoe and Cameron are my closest friends from grad school and have also recently fallen in love with each other. It's pretty cute—in the manner of adorable puppy and kitten calendars—so to compensate for being the third wheel, I order a double gin and tonic. Then I order some fries. French fries would be my dying meal if I were ever to experience the misfortune of a death sentence, and after four drinks, I am completely powerless to resist them. So much for those three hundred calories I've just burned. I tell my friends that I'm waiting to hear from Rob after his first day on a porn shoot.

"That's a weird one," says Zoe.

"Yes, my boyfriend is currently filming close-ups of people *doing it,*" I slur.

"It's a bit out of the norm," she says. Cam shrugs his shoulders. Zoe darts him a wide-eyed "Thank God I'm not dealing with her issues!" look.

Good for fucking you guys in your honeymoon phase, I think, and order another double. My night takes a turn for the better when a frat boy in a hockey jersey climbs up on stage and starts earnestly singing Tracy Chapman's "Fast Car." Cam has to usher me out of the audience because my laughter is inappropriate. Sometime later, I wake up on my couch. I hobble to the kitchen and chug a glass of water. It's three in the morning. I call Rob.

"Hello," he says. I can tell I've woken him.

"Hey, sorry, I went out and had one too many gin and tonics," I say. "How did it go?"

"It was okay. Do you want to talk about it in the morning?"

"It *is* the morning. Yeah, okay. Can you give me a preview?"

"Well, you'll never believe it, but we ended up filming a foursome and one of the girls was a squirter. It was pretty crazy. I literally had to jump away with the camera not to get hit."

He sounds fully awake now, stoked. Like it was some cool adventure. Despite the numbing qualities of the booze, my stomach does one of those Tower Drop plunges that comes from feeling left out.

He tells me that they filmed at a hotel in the Valley. The room was crammed with two film crews—the actual porn crew and Robbie's crew—as well as four porn stars screwing the dickens out of each other. The heat was of a tropical degree; the smells pungent as gardenia, only different. Post–squirter scene, the whole room was drenched—bedcover, carpets, curtains—all sopping wet.

"So it's real," I say.

"I don't think you can fake what I saw."

"Was it a turn-on?" I ask. "Never mind, don't answer that. I guess this could have waited until tomorrow after all. I love you. Call you in the morning."

"I love you too, more than anything."

The next day I wake to the sound of rain splattering on the window. The first thing I think of, yet again, is an acrobatic squirting fuckathon. I'm visualizing sex constantly, which seems like it should be more enjoyable. I guess this is how perverts feel, or perhaps just all men? Then I register my dull aching head and realize I'm late. I have an appointment with my acupuncturist, Tanya Gee. (Yes, I have an acupuncturist, as well as an herbalist and a psychic. My mother is what you would call an alternative medicine aficionado.) I drag myself to the bathroom to splash water on my face, which looks less than fresh.

Although I plan to hide my hangover and the fact that I've lost my mind, it takes Tanya about two-point-five seconds to see through me. I am clearly extremely poor at subterfuge. That said, my poor state of mental health is about as covert as Britney Spears was on the day she shaved her head.

"Okay, what's going on?" T says, as I recline on the table.

"Robbie's shooting porn," I say. "Well, actually he's shooting *people* shooting porn. It's for a reality TV show."

"And it's bothering you?"

"I drank enough gin to anesthetize an elephant last night."

"Why do you think that is?"

"We had a dumb fight because he lied to me about watching porn, then he was off filming it. I'm not having an easy time with it."

"That's unfortunate timing," she says.

"Am I nuts to be uncomfortable with this?"

"No," she says. "But you trust Robbie, don't you?"

"Yes," I blubber.

"Then you have to trust that even though he may get a thrill from what he's filming, he's still coming home to you."

"I guess that's true."

"Trust Robbie, Em. You two are good for each other. Trust yourself and try to let go of the details."

All the while, Tanya has been sticking me with tiny needles. She dims the lights and turns on some soothing music—*Ocean Waves at Sunset, Volume Four*, or some shit. I know she's right; I do have to trust Robbie. After all, unbeknownst to Tanya, we're engaged. I certainly have to find a better way of dealing with my discomfort than mainlining gin.

"See you in a little while," T whispers as she shuts the door, leaving me in darkness with the crashing sounds of the Pacific.

Just what I need, the gushing sounds of water. Great.

If I knew then what I know now, I'd wonder why I couldn't ditch my compulsive thoughts about what Robbie was filming and carry on with my day. But I suppose anyone who's ever been stuck on something in a relationship knows how obsessive thoughts can reel you in and wring you out. Maybe you know how it feels to fixate over the way your boyfriend checked someone out in a restaurant. Perhaps you once found yourself stewing when your partner Facebook-friended a tumultuous ex. Jealous thoughts, founded or unfounded, can bubble up unpredictably and boil relentlessly until the pot's charred dry. With a healthy dose of hindsight, I've discovered that my initial qualms with Robbie filming porn were rooted in feeling possessive and worrying about his expectations of me.

Monogamy, defined as having one sexual partner, presumes a kind of ownership—I give myself to you, body and soul, and you give yourself to me, *yada yada*. But if we subscribe to this idea, as Robbie and I did, then exactly how much of our significant other's body and soul do we get? How much do we want to give? It's my understanding that within monogamy, there are many interpretations, and it's up to the couples to define. Being sexually exclusive these days, after all, isn't always cut-and-dry.

For example, does sending a Twitter picture of your junk to someone other than your spouse constitute a breach in monogamy? Is kissing someone else but not having sex with them okay? How about strip clubs—look but don't touch? Lap dances—look and get touched but don't touch? What about watching porn? If pornography is okay in your monogamy agreement (it is not kosher in everyone's contract; for example, Dr. Phil's or maybe your god's, depending), then does it matter what kind of images? Say, everything but bestiality goes? What about how much is consumed? Or whether you watch it together? On the other hand, is what you or your lover watches simply off limits, not up for discussion? There are many ways to go. Often these aren't terms we define until contracts are breached; we'd prefer not to talk about these niggling details. And sometimes we don't know how we feel until, well, shit happens.

Personally, I do not believe that watching porn is cheating. I think there's a distinction between watching something on a screen and participating in the flesh. Nonetheless, once upon a time, my intellectual understanding and my emotional responses didn't add up. I didn't expect the waves of jealousy that crashed over me when I thought about my fiancé filming porn, which somehow *felt* one step closer than just watching it (not that I liked to think about that either). These people were real. I felt possessive. I didn't like to think about him being attracted to anybody else (in this case, hot, naked women at his workplace)—even if I believed there was a vast difference between attraction and acting on something. Consciously or not, romantic and naïve to be sure, I preferred the Jane Austen–esque fantasy that I held exclusive rights to his attraction. Apparently, I had some ownership issues I hadn't addressed. Up they bubbled.

At the time, I also felt angry and deceived when Robbie wasn't completely frank about this particular porn preference. His lie (though an understandable and natural response to my discomfort) was an easier thing to be mad about than facing what was really bothering me. One can interpret that my snappy judgment about squirting—*that can't possibly be real!*—was triggered by my own insecurity. Robbie had a desire I couldn't fulfill, and I worried I couldn't live up to his expectations.

In the past, my way of dealing with my discomfort around porn was to separate myself from it. Porn was lowbrow, stupid, and vulgar. I figured I was more . . . sophisticated, educated, refined, whatnot. In truth, however, I envied the sexually brazen world presented by porn, a world where nobody seemed awkward or inhibited. I was nothing like the girls on screen, neither physically nor seemingly emotionally. And those girls were what guys—my guy—fantasized about.

In these moments, it didn't matter that I was engaged to a man who loved me for who I was. I was too deeply immersed in my own fiction. I like to think that I'm someone who can separate fact from fiction, but I guess there's a reason I'm not captivated by werewolves and vampires. When it came to porn, I clearly had a hard time with the concept of fantasy. Porn is fantasy! Fun! Not a set of expectations for women or men, goes the rationale—seems simple enough. Robbie never wanted or expected me to represent every aspect of his desires. *In fact, the pervasive societal rub is that girlfriends and wives acting like porn stars is often the furthest thing from what guys want.* Nonetheless, I felt compared. Is that what he wants me to act like, look like, do? Wow, I must suck (or, if you will, not suck nearly enough). Notice how I couldn't stop looking through the lens of what Robbie thought, which isn't very self-empowered at all, actually.

Alas, if I knew then what I know now, I'd be able to see all of these things more rationally. I'd also be able to consider how Googling local sex shops to see if there were any upcoming workshops on squirting might have been a more productive way to go. Or I could have procured myself a copy of *The Secret of Great G-Spot Orgasms and Female Ejaculation* by Tristan Taorimo, one of the more feminist-minded porn producers out there. It's not lost on me now that for someone to whom this act doesn't come naturally, so to speak, mastering it requires relaxation and trust. The emotional abandonment precedes the physical. Apt metaphors for a girl who was feeling all clammed up.

Come to think of it, squirting would have been a great exercise.

For now I lie rigid, needles sunk in my forehead and wrists, waiting for Tanya Gee's egg timer to signal that twenty minutes of repose are up. In fact, I'm about as relaxed as an '80s executive after snorting a caterpillar line of cocaine. Anxious, irrational, hungover, all I can think about is going home, closing the blinds, and climbing back into bed. Today I'm thankful for the lack of sun, happy to disappear like change down the grate on this dreary, forgettable Vancouver day.

CHAPTER 2

GONZO

Through a layer of beige smog, I touch down at LAX. Two years of long distance finally ditched north of the border. I tried to sleep away the three-hour flight, but my brain was too busy computing the gravity of this plane ride: I am about to move in with the man I will marry.

Up until now, my life commitments have been semipermanent. A degree here, a transcontinental trip there. But this is bigger. It's the first time I'm letting a relationship dictate the shape of my life, my where-abouts. We have never lived together. Now we will share a roof presumably, well, forever, unless we become one of those couples with separate abodes. Anyway, my single life has been crammed into two very large suitcases in the cargo hold and several boxes of books arriving via UPS.

I rise from my seat and wait with the stomping herd of passengers to disembark. Despite my anxiousness, I smile politely at an elderly woman, clad entirely in beige, dawdling in the aisle. *I've waited this long, what's another two minutes, Grandma?* In the terminal, I walk briskly to

Customs with my three-year visa in hand. They nod me through like a veritable American, and I beeline to the baggage carousel.

Since that miserable day when I lay depressed and hungover on the acupuncture table, I've adjusted my attitude a smidge. I'm no longer chugging gin (every night). And I'm attempting the "letting go" stance Dr. Tanya Gee encouraged. So when Robbie informed me last night that he'd be filming porn today when I arrived, and thus unable to collect me at LAX, I said, "No problem!" So here I am, making my way solo through the sliding doors, out into the balmy, polluted Los Angeles air. The smell is nostalgic of childhood vacations, except I'm not going to Disneyland. I live here. My heavily laden airport cart bumps and heaves as I wheel it to the shuttle pickup. The cute wool-blend dress and heeled loafers I decided to wear today now seem like less of a good idea. Yet again, an attempt to be fashion forward has me perspiring like Gerard Depardieu.

With my crap loaded in the van, I snag a window seat. From my many visits, I already have my general bearings. We speed along the 105 Freeway to the 110, pass the small cluster of buildings that comprise downtown, and merge onto the 101. As usual, trash lines the roadside. LA, in my experience, is filthy and full of juxtapositions—vegan cafés next to Jack in the Boxes, hybrids cruise alongside Hummers. I like the irony, if not the exhaust. We exit the freeway in Hollywood. His apartment is located between the multimillion-dollar homes above Franklin Avenue and the seedy vibe of east Hollywood Boulevard. Cheap motels blink promises of ADULT VIDEOS. How on point they now seem. I'm the van's third stop as we enter Los Feliz. We turn down Russell Ave. Thin palms loom high in the muted blue sky. I spot the tall white columns outside his butter-yellow apartment—our apartment, that is. The driver slows to a stop and then helps me get my bags to the curb. I haul my suitcases up onto the sidewalk and through the metal gate. Our unit is the front, bottom-floor apartment on the left side of the small complex. The yard is bright green with coarse tropical grass. Red and pink roses bloom in the flowerbeds down the center pathway and alongside the perimeter fence. I lean in and smell them. Outside the apartment door, a case of empty Tecate cans sits on a dirty folding lawn chair; it's been there since I visited two months ago. I turn my key in the lock.

The door opens up to a large rectangular living room. I kick off my heels and dump my heavy bags with a thud. Floor-to-ceiling windows covered by dusty venetian blinds cast a hazy light. I've been here before. I painted the walls "lion" beige with Robbie and his roommate when they moved in. But this is the first time I've looked at the space as my own. I make a mental note to shop for curtains. Furniture is sparse— an L-shaped couch, a TV resting on IKEA cubes, and a coffee table. In stocking feet, I walk left into the dining room where a card table and chairs make a sunny eating space. The narrow kitchen opens off the dining room. A few dishes are piled in the sink. I brush aside the thought that Robbie didn't leave things clean for me. I open the fridge—beer and condiments. It's a single man's home. I walk the rest of the apartment, taking in my new life. I investigate the evidence like I used to as a teenage babysitter—refrigerated pot roasts and junk drawers revealing a history. I pull my damp dress over my head and drop it on the couch as I pass. Two bedrooms and a bathroom constitute the rest of the apartment. The back room is dark and empty since Robbie's film school roommate left to move in with his girlfriend. I peer out the small window to the courtyard where a fountain gurgles. We'll have a guest bed here, maybe a desk. The Pepto Bismol pink–tiled bathroom separates the two bedrooms. Robbie's room looks out to the front yard. The bed is made, a small pile of clothes strewn atop it. I pick up a pale blue button-down shirt. It smells like Robbie. I breathe into it—Tide, Old Spice, a hint of his sweat, home. More dusty venetians obscure the rose beds outside. I pull the cord and sunlight blares in. I think I'll like it here.

I haul my bags into the bedroom and return to the living room couch, where I collapse. I plan to rise in exactly five minutes and start unpacking. My mind is already tidying, mopping floors, and making a mental list of furniture we will need to acquire. But instead of doing anything, I fall instantly into a deep, delicious sleep.

Two hours later, I wake to dim evening light and the sound of keys. I sit up as Robbie comes through the door. He looks distracted. Actually, he looks like he forgot I was going to be here.

"Hi!" he says, registering my presence and clearly attempting to put on the cheer.

"Hi there," I say. "I fell asleep. But I'm here. How was it?" I rise from the couch to give him a kiss but he ducks my advance.

"Let me shower first," he says. "You'll thank me later."

"Okay," I say, feeling slightly shunted and wondering since when we shower before kissing. He didn't even remark on my being in nothing but tights and a bra. Chilly from sleep, I pull my dress back on and follow him into the bedroom. He strips off his clothes and throws them in the hamper. "Are you okay?" I ask.

"Yeah, it was pretty insane. I'll tell you all about it, but I need to get clean. Two minutes."

He goes to the bathroom and turns on the water. I retreat to the kitchen, feeling increasingly anxious and frankly a little rejected. What happened today? I occupy myself with making an impromptu snack—mildly stale corn chips and an avocado mashed into some jarred salsa. I grab two Coronas and place it all on the coffee table. Robbie comes out with a towel wrapped around his waist. He sits with his legs splayed open on the couch, turquoise terry cloth barely covering him. I have the urge to jump him, but I sense it's not the moment. Usually he can't keep his hands off me when we've been apart. But I can tell his suggestive stance is unintentional. His mind is clearly occupied and not with thoughts of me.

"So?" I say.

"How much detail do you want?" he asks.

"All of it, like we agreed. Full disclosure."

"Okay," he says and begins to unravel the events of the day.

He tells me they were back in the San Fernando Valley at another unsuspecting hotel. The director, a burly black guy who goes by the name Nine, was in the living room of the suite readying camera equipment. There were four porn stars on set—three muscular black dudes in the bedroom and a slim brunette having her makeup done in the bathroom. The bedroom was a tight space, made more cramped by Nine's assistant, Valaria, a Montreal porn star who was looking to break into the LA scene. She'd flown in that morning to shadow Nine for a week and make introductions. Her role today was to hold a small handheld camera and get additional perspectives on the action.

"Did you know the lead girl?" I ask, immediately wondering if he was confronting an online fantasy in the flesh.

"No," he shakes his head. "She was pretty worn-down-looking though. Kind of hooker hot."

"Oh," I say, conjuring an image of Courtney Love–meets–Kit De Luca. Is that a good thing? I can't tell. Robbie goes on with his story.

He filmed Valaria as she fiddled with her camera in the corner of the room. She was young, curvaceous, dressed in shorts and a cleavage-revealing yellow top. The three black guys started teasing her.

"You going to be joining us?" one asked. She giggled and shook her head no.

"You sure about that?" said another and walked up close to her, almost touching. He backed her tauntingly toward the bed.

"Hey, stop," she said, and the other two crowded over her so that she clumsily fell backward. Was this mock protest? Robbie didn't know. He kept rolling. Nine was still in the other room. One of the guys started undoing her shorts. Another pulled her underwear down.

"Wait a minute," I interject. "I don't want to throw around the *R* word, but this sounds like coercion."

"I know," he says. "It was borderline. I felt awkward. But she was also smiling, laughing."

I raise my eyebrows at Robbie. He continues.

The dude started going down on her. Valaria kept protesting and laughing as they took turns on her. Nine sauntered into the room and rolled his eyes.

"Quit it, Valaria!" he said, and the guys moved off her. She picked up her handheld, which she'd discarded on the bed, and pulled her shorts up. The female lead entered the room naked except for her stilettos and makeup. She shot a bitchy look at Valaria. Nine dialed Talent Testing Service on the room phone so that the four performers could verify their STD-negative results. They get tested every twenty-two days, Robbie explained, and call in before every porn shoot. With the *all clean* go-ahead, Nine began to roll. Robbie kept filming too, attempting the intricate task of avoiding erections and penetration in a small room with four people fucking. Michel, *Webdream*'s director, had instructed him that any such footage would be useless in the final cut, in accordance with prime-time guidelines. The performers went straight to it. Fucking the girl vaginally, anally, and in the mouth at once. Then one of the guys turned his attention to Valaria again.

"Come on, sexy, get in here," he said. Valaria looked to Nine for guidance, but his head was obscured behind the camera.

"Yeah, baby girl," another encouraged. She asked Nine if she could join in. He didn't answer. Instead, he commanded some direction to the female lead, who leaned her cheek into the bedspread and raised her ass in the air to give him a better angle. Valaria looked back and forth between Nine and the guys. She slipped off her clothes and climbed on the bed. Nine continued to film, unflinchingly. The two girls started making out with each other while two of the guys did them from behind. The third guy stood on the bed to have his dick sucked by both of them. All three of the guys were more interested in Valaria. The lead female looked pissed. Nine muttered to himself, indicating his disapproval. But he didn't ask Valaria to stop.

Robbie moved around the bed, trying to stay out of the way. The three guys rotated on and off the mattress, inadvertently brushing sweaty body parts against Robbie as they passed. The female lead directed her performance at Robbie, who held the biggest camera. She made fuck-me, *oohing, ahhing* faces. The room grew sweltering. When it was time for the money shot, Nine told Valaria to get out of the scene, and the four main performers moved to the living room of the suite. The female lead kneeled on the carpet while the guys took turns cumming on her face. For the third money shot, Robbie moved to find another angle, barely dodging a stream of ejaculate. He made a mental note not to wear shorts next time.

The girl turned to Robbie's camera, and with cum dripping down her face she began chatting about her weekend plans. He couldn't tell whether she was genuinely oblivious, accustomed to making small talk while covered in jizz, or just fucking with him. Eventually, she got off her knees and went to the bathroom to wash her face. Nine wrote checks to the four performers and everyone left, leaving him and Valaria alone.

"What the hell were you thinking?" Nine said. He unleashed on her, rebuking her for being completely unprofessional, telling her that she was an idiot for risking giving the other performers STDs. He said she'd completely blown her chance, then went to the room phone and asked the concierge to call a cab. He was sending her to LAX. She started crying, grabbed her bags, and stormed out of the room.

"Did you follow her?" I ask. My hand is jittery holding my beer, so I put it down.

"No, we didn't know whether to stay with her or Nine. We stayed with him because we only had one camera."

"Wow," I say. "I can't believe he didn't stop her from having sex with them."

"I know," Robbie says.

We sit in silence for a minute looking at each other. He's still in his towel, legs tipped open. But sex is now the last thing on my mind. Nor am I remotely hungry anymore. I feel angry. But for whom? For Valaria, I guess. My discomfort surges through me like lightning looking for an exit.

"How old is Valaria?"

"Nineteen, maybe. Twenty?"

"Do you think she really wanted to do any of that, or was she just trying to get noticed?"

"I don't know. It was weird the way the guys went down on her. I really couldn't tell what she wanted."

"It sounds so fucking sketchy. This is exactly the kind of thing I expected and yet didn't want to hear."

"I know. I guess she's a porn star back in Montreal. So it's not the first time she's fucked on film."

"Does that make it better?" I blurt, not intending for it to come out like a slap in the face.

"I don't know." He shrugs, looking defeated.

"Then there's the girl having three guys cum on her face . . ." I shudder. I always have trouble getting my mind around how any woman is up for that. Robbie stares into space, giving no reaction. "What do you think about 'face shots'?" I ask, enunciating the term like I'm reading it from the dictionary for the first time.

He looks at me tentatively. "Well, it wasn't against her will," he says. "She was getting paid. That's just the way this type of scene usually ends."

Why do guys want to see that? Does he think it's hot? I want to ask. But I don't really want to fight with him about whether face shots are degrading. I want to remain on the same page about how messed up the day was. "Are you going to be okay with filming this kind of thing all the time?" I ask instead.

"I don't know," he says. "I think I can separate myself from it. But it's definitely more hard-core than I expected."

"I feel weird knowing that's where you were today," I say.

"I understand." He puts a hand on my knee and I have the sudden urge to shake it off, as if he's done something wrong. "Do you want me to quit?" he says, reading some portion of my thoughts.

"No," I say emphatically, "that's not the solution." But what is? I still don't want him to quit because this makes me uncomfortable. The world won't be any different whether he records what happens in the Valley or not. Surely I can find a corner of myself in which to stash my conflicting emotions. Or better yet, resolve them once and for all. "Do you think their parents know what they do? I mean, how do you think they got into this world?" I say.

"I don't know," he says. "Michel doesn't ask questions like that. The show's angle is chronicling where they want to go in their careers. This plotline is more about Nine trying to become a big-shot gonzo producer."

"What's 'gonzo' again?" I ask, feeling like an idiot. *Money shots, gonzo—this new language is as comprehensive to me as Russian written in Brail.*

"It's what we filmed today. No plotline, handheld camera footage with lots of close-ups, straight to the hard-core stuff with hardly any buildup."

"Ah, right, just what every girl *loves*."

"What?" Robbie says, missing my sarcasm.

"I mean, most of us like a little foreplay before sex, not to mention before getting fucked every which way by three guys. I'm just saying—*that's how I like a gang bang to go down,*" I say, attempting a joke. Robbie cracks a sympathetic smile.

"It's not meant to be reality, Em."

"I guess not," I concur. "But if you're a teenage boy getting your sex education online, you might think that's what girls want. And girls might think that's how guys want them to behave."

"Come on, I think most of us can read between the lines," he says.

"You'd be surprised."

"Are we going to start man-hating now?" he says teasingly. "I turned out okay, didn't I?"

"We'll see what you're like after a few months of this," I joke back. My voice comes out like chipped ice. I realize that I am sitting with my legs and arms crossed—a highly guarded position, according to Body Language 101. I uncross my arms and take a deep breath. Cool summer air wafts through the open window. The sun has descended. A car blaring hip-hop passes outside.

Robbie watches me closely, aware of our unintentional face-off. He stands and holds out his hand to me. "Okay, this isn't the introduction I'd planned. Can I take you to dinner?"

"Yes," I say exhaling. "Please, let's."

Across the wrought-iron table at a neighborhood French bistro we do our best to put the topic aside. But I can't help replaying my imagined version, as I suspect Robbie's head is full of literal images. We smile at each other. Discuss whether to order the Sancerre or the Chablis. Settle on sharing the crab cakes to start.

"Any questions before you order?" our server asks. He's cute, a twentysomething who is either part French or just an aspiring Hollywood actor playing the part.

Any questions? Oh yes, so many. You see, my fiancé here has been filming porn all day. What do you think of porn? You like it, right? I guess most guys do. Okay, then what do you think of face shots specifically? Degrading or not? I lean toward yes, but my fiancé here says that as long as it's consensual, it's fair play. But nobody knows or really monitors the exact politics of consent behind what we're watching on screen, do they? Like what happened today. This poor girl got fired . . .

"Mademoiselle?" he says, awaiting my answer. I nod my head no and say, "I'll have the hanger steak, please. Medium rare."

Face shots are easy to take offense to. The symbolism is blunt. Thus, unsurprisingly, the proliferation of cumming on a woman's face in XXX forms the crux of many a feminist antiporn argument, an argument I have wielded before. How many real-world women and men truly enjoy this—how shall we say it—display of affection? I can't say. What I do know is that a glance at the world of hard-core porn informs us that all women today like having cum run through our carefully applied mascara. Right, ladies? We just love it! This farce used to bother me quite a bit.

Over time, I've come to see things differently and I no longer get my back up about this staple porn cliché. Why? I have an easier time comprehending that while this may not be my particular fantasy, it's someone else's, and not mine to judge. Face shots in porn are part of a script enacted by paid performers. And what folks choose to reenact in the privacy of their bedrooms is entirely up to them. But don't get me wrong—there is no question in my mind that Internet porn has made this act more prolific, if not even a mainstream expectation, among young men and women today. I'm not the only one who's noticed this trend.

A few years ago a website called MakeLoveNotPorn was developed to address how porn affects bedroom expectations, and to offer an alternative conversation. Cindy Gallop formed this website in 2008 as a reaction to the lack of diversity she saw in hard-core porn. In her sixties, Cindy generally dates younger men—mostly twentysomethings from the Gen Y cohort. She experienced firsthand how young men who've grown up consuming Internet porn take certain realities for granted. For example, this oft-demonstrated notion that all women simply adore having jism ejaculated onto their face. Cindy considers herself pro-sex and pro-porn. Her take is this: Some men and women take pleasure in this act. Some do not. It's a personal thing. Nevertheless, the porn world presents a version of sexual reality that comes with biases we should be aware of. She believes that we can benefit from being conscious of how the widespread consumption of XXX is affecting our behavior. I couldn't agree more.

But at the time, I was just becoming aware of what happens in mainstream porn. And by "becoming aware," I mean being slapped in the face by a porn tsunami. My fiancé was quite suddenly filming real men cumming on real women's faces. I was clinging to a rickety fence—an old, feminist notion of what was degrading—in a forceful tide. I obsessed about what the performers, particularly the women, whom I identified with more closely, were going through. Especially when Robbie was returning home with stories like the one about Valaria. There were also the general things about porn content to consider. Are face shots inherently degrading? And then there were the politics of the way porn was being made. Last, there was my own world of sexual prejudices to confront. I was feeling uncomfortable in my own skin, insecure and prudish compared to the brazen world of anything-goes porn. I felt self-righteous for Valaria. Piteous of the girl with cum dripping down her face. Angry at Nine (and porn producers in general). I felt mistrustful of *Webdreams'* agenda, and of Robbie for playing witness to it all.

But I couldn't see any of this clearly then. Not yet. I could only see the pink center of the cut of meat before me on my dinner plate. And I had no appetite. I looked to my fiancé across the table from me. He lifted a forkful of Sole à la Meunière to his mouth. I could only think about what else his eyes had feasted on that day.

CHAPTER 3

SHAVED

This morning we finally find our mojo. After porn talk, dinner, and wine last night, we were both too weary to consummate our newly engaged life together. This morning I managed to tune it all out. Now we're lying entwined in our sun-dappled bed in a state of postcoital bliss. I run my fingers through Robbie's facial hair, tracing his chin, grazing my fingernails over his shaved head. He leans into my touch.

"Sorry I'm so burly for you," Robbie says, referring to his longer-than-normal beard and unshaved neck. "I meant to get around to that."

"I don't mind; I've been a little lax on the grooming myself," I say. I too meant to spend more time with a razor before arriving. Moving obliterated two weeks of my life. While I'm not exactly Amazonian, I'm no porn star either. I should have exerted more effort given the company my fiancé has been keeping. After all, I know how it feels to have my grooming efforts up for judgment.

In my early twenties, I had a brief, pathetic fling with a friend of mine whom I'll call Trevor. As is predictable when sleeping with friends, things ended poorly. I can't remember if we stopped seeing each other after the incident when I fell off a couch and hit my head, hard, on a coffee table, and he responded by laughing and refilling his wineglass, or if it was after the time he brought another girl to the sushi restaurant where I bartended and made out with her at the bar. Either way, it was over before it clambered off the ground.

Trevor and I drank copious amounts of red wine together and brought out the worst in each other. I'd been hanging around him because I was trying to get with his roommate when Trevor and I rolled, drunk, into bed together. He'd had a crush on me, he'd confessed, and though willing to bed me, he had a sizable chip on his shoulder for being sloppy seconds. So it was that on one special night of our courtship, lying naked together, he asked, "What's with the bohemian hair?" Unfortunately, he wasn't referring to my long brown tresses. He nodded toward my nether regions. "You and Hilary [a mutual friend of ours whom he'd also fooled around with], you're all Joni Mitchell."

I didn't know what to be more offended by, the attack on my cha cha (yes, I sometimes like to refer to my vagina as a whimsical Latin dance) or the fact that he was comparing my girly parts to my friend's. I'd always been a groomer—you wouldn't have found me rocking a German bikini line by the seaside—but I guess I had more hair down there than some. To be sure, the next day I spent quality time in the bathroom with wax strips and Nair. In an attempt to be extra thorough, I found out what happens when you leave Nair on too long. So thank you, Trevor, for that week I spent rubbing Polysporin on my seared ass.

When I met Robbie a few years later, I'd recovered from the burn of embarrassment and generally maintained the same groomed, but not totally bare, appearance. Until one evening when Robbie was visiting Vancouver, and he suggested we do a little couples trimming together. With a little cajoling and a fair bit of champagne, I allowed him to remove all evidence I was a grown woman.

"My vagina had chemo!" were the words that flew out of my mouth. As imaginable, that was kind of a fun-stopper. What I didn't say was that I felt vulnerable, exposed. I guess I was a little Joni Mitchell after all— both in my au naturel preference and in my high-pitched sensitivity.

Not too much has changed since then, though I did intend to be more prepared for this lovers' reunion. Clearly, with the promise of "together forever," I have already let myself go a tad. The good news is that Robbie isn't exactly what you'd call picky. I could likely grow a moustache and he'd still get it on with me. Nevertheless, I shouldn't take apathy too far—it's insidious, I hear. And we haven't even walked down the aisle yet. For the moment, he has to go to work.

"One of my film school buddies is having a party tonight if we want to go. It's on the west side, so maybe Hilary can bring you, and I'll meet you there after Malibu?" Robbie says as he gets out of bed and pulls a shirt over his head. He is off to another shoot today. I'll have the day to myself to settle in.

"Sure, I'll ask her." A blessing in my move to LA is that Hilary (yes, of the Woodstock-era comparison) lives here. She's a close friend from Montreal, and I'm relieved to know one person other than Robbie in this overcrowded city. I sit up on the bed and swing my legs over the side. "Okay if I make space in the closet?"

"Of course, it's your home," he says and leans in for a kiss. "I'll text you the address. See you tonight." The screen door clacks shut. I am alone again. Which is fine. I've grown accustomed to solitude after the last few years.

I decide to settle into my environment—to add a little of myself and remove a layer of grit from our home. First, I hang clothes and fill a couple of dresser drawers. Then I pull out a broom and sweep dust bunnies out of the corners and from under the bed. I'm not always the neatest person, but I can't stand a dirty floor. Before long, I'm in the full swing of a ritual cleaning, pulling covers off of living room cushions and tossing them in the wash. We might as well start out April-fresh. I power up my laptop and turn on some reggae. The sunshine and breeze wafting through the open windows seem to support my new start.

Later that afternoon, as I pull the dry cushion covers off the clothesline in the courtyard, I feel good about life. Remarkably, I've only had the occasional fleeting thought about whom or what Robbie is off filming. A success of grand proportions compared to my former OCD, I'd say. After yesterday, I decided I simply have to compartmentalize his job and go with the flow. I have to not think, for thinking will be my demise.

Hilary has agreed to pick me up and drive to West Hollywood. My sweaty rat's-nest hair and California Raisins t-shirt aren't going to impress anyone. I don a silk top and dressy shorts with heels, put on some mascara and lip gloss, and blow-dry my hair. I'm looking very LA, I figure, when Hilary rolls up in her beat-up Mercedes. Hil works at American Apparel, where they seem to dole out these vintage cars to their employees like condoms at a campus health clinic. I could probably use a car, but Robbie and I will share his old Hyundai for now. The truth is, I'm relieved to have to depend on rides. I'm a bad driver. The gist of it is, I have zero spatial relationships, and I maneuver as if in a bumper car, much to the dismay of other drivers. Needless to say, parallel parking is a problem. As well, five-lane highways make me instinctively close my eyes in fear. The Google map feature "avoid freeways" is my friend. It takes me twice as long as anyone else to get somewhere. In LA, that is a long time.

"Hey, lady! You're dressy," Hilary says, and hops out of the driver seat to give me a big hug on the street. My pumps bring me just shy of her five feet six inches and land my cheek in her masses of curly brown hair. She's wearing jeans, boat shoes, and a men's wool cardigan over a bra-revealing tank top, but somehow making it look casually sexy rather than frumpy. Whereas if I put on that outfit, I'd look homeless.

"Should I change?" I ask.

"No, no," she says. "It's a party, right? I just worked from home today and never bothered. I'll put some eyeliner on when we get there." We pull away and enter our usual deluge of catch-up conversation. She drives with one knee propped up like she's watching late-night TV, not changing lanes. Whereas I drive like I'm being open-fired on. I fill her in on my visa situation and she gives me the highlights of her love life. She's been in an on-again-off-again replay with this guy Tucker for a couple of years. They're on again. Nevertheless, at a bar the week prior, he was visibly checking out a model-slash-actress. This breed of woman, she tells me, distresses normal girls trying to date in LA, as *E. coli* distresses produce. It's actually nice to know this type of thing bothers Hilary. Not everyone is as blasé as they sometimes seem.

"So, yeah, same old," she says. "Whose party are we going to anyway?"

"It's Simon's—he's a friend of Robbie's from film school. I should know a couple people."

"And Robbie's meeting us there?"

"Yeah, he's filming a threesome at a Malibu mansion."

"Ah, right."

"Yup! This is my new life."

"You seem mellow about it."

"I'm taking the high road."

"Well, if anyone can handle it, it's you guys after all you've been through. I don't think I'd particularly like Tucker filming porn if I can't even handle him checking out the next Megan Fox."

I don't care to revisit how I'm not always dealing with my situation gracefully. Instead, I say, "I think this is the place," as we pull up to a 1940s-looking apartment building with fire escapes down the exterior. We find parking on the street and climb to the fourth floor. I quickly realize I was wrong about knowing anyone other than Simon, who politely introduces us around and deposits us in the living room with glasses of red wine.

So far, the party consists of a group of people smoking pot in a bedroom and some guys watching basketball on the couch next to us. Thankfully, Hilary is here. Not only so we can entertain ourselves, but also because, unlike me, she's a whiz at small talk. She's also a basketball fan and quickly pipes in on the action, making what I can only assume are apt comments, whereas I say things like, "Get it!" at inopportune times. I also note that everyone else seems to be dressed for winter. Did I miss the sweater party memo? Several people have remarked on the unseasonably cold July weather, which to me, since I grew up in an igloo, is sultry. I might as well be wearing a Hooters uniform in this crowd of hipster cardigans. I tuck heartily in to the chips and gulp my wine, wondering how long it will take for Robbie to get here and loan me a sweater. He said he'd be here by eight-thirty or nine.

At eleven o'clock, we are ready to leave when Robbie shows up with Michel, the director of the show. The party is happening now, and Robbie makes an entrance into the crammed kitchen where everyone is making cocktails and fetching beers from the fridge. Clearly, these are his people. A girl in a fedora hat pushes through the crowd to Robbie and gives him a huge hug.

Once, in a moment of so-called relationship maturity, Robbie and

I talked about which of our respective fellow grad students we found attractive. At the time, it hadn't bothered me when he'd described a girl he thought was cute. Now I'm experiencing why such conversations are destined to backfire. Was it her: Fedora Girl? Was she at that party where he "passed out on the couch" one night and didn't check in? *Don't go there, brain*, I plead. I am here now; we are together. We made it through the shit. I feel comparative, on guard. Robbie's banter with everyone makes me miss my grad school friends in Vancouver. *I had a life but I left it for you, Bucko . . .* my ego prattles on.

A brief word about long-distance relationships: Like most people who enter these types of precarious arrangements, we didn't know if we could make it; we only knew we wanted to try. So we kept communication lines humming. We talked through our fears and anxieties over "Anytime North America" plans. We made promises. We assured each other we'd raise a white flag if we changed our minds or failed. But as anyone who's ever lived through a long-distance relationship knows, no amount of trust can completely quell the anxieties that come with the terrain. Suspicions seep in. I like to think that a dash of jealousy in a relationship means that we care. Another interpretation is that we're shit-our-pants petrified of betrayal—we've all seen it happen, or we've lived it. We feel even more vulnerable over distance, and we are, so we gravitate to the armor of doubt to protect us. The seasoned irony of loving and being loved, however, is that we must trust one another to get anywhere. This is a rather delicate equilibrium.

Has two years apart solidified my convictions or rendered me psycho and volatile? Am I primed for success or disaster? I'm not sure. Just as I'm veering into the oncoming lane, Robbie leans in and kisses me. "Sorry we're so late," he whispers in my ear, "you look hot." Then he hugs Hilary and introduces us to Michel.

"How did the shoot go?" I ask.

"Good for us, but bad for them," Michel says. Simon, a couple of other guys, and Fedora Girl close in around us. Simon pipes up.

"You're directing the porn show Robbie was telling us about?"

"Yes," Michel grins. "That's us."

"How was it bad for them?" I ask.

"The scene was with two girls and a guy, and he couldn't stay hard," says Michel.

"That's an important skill for a porn star," Hilary says.

"No kidding," says Fedora Girl. "What did they do?"

"The girls just did a lesbian scene."

"I'm curious. What are these women like?" Fedora Girl asks. Suddenly I'm thrilled to have her there, instigating questions so that I don't have to.

"Yeah, what's their vibe?" I second.

"It really depends," says Michel. "Some of them do it on the side of other things, like one girl today was in law school. Others are really serious about their porn careers. And I guess we see some girls who, how do you say, Robbie? Seem a little . . ." Michel gives a so-so hand gesture that I assume means "kind of off."

"One of the girls today seemed pretty hungover or maybe still on something," Robbie says.

"So it's a mix," Michel concurs. "A lot of them have a similar look—implants, tanned, acrylic nails, lots of makeup, shaved bare," Michel gives us the details we want.

"Well who isn't bare these days," Fedora Girl says. Michel shrugs.

I instantly fear that my pubic hair is hanging out of my short shorts. It couldn't be that out of control down there—could it? Christ, who doesn't trim up before wearing short shorts? I don't.

"Yeah, pubic hair, who has it . . ." I stutter, realizing I have to change the topic by the ABORT eyes Hilary is making at me. "So how much do porn stars make, Michel?" I ask with news-anchor formality. I'm quite certain my cheeks are now the same tint as my berry lip gloss. I focus on Michel, hoping everybody will just assume I'm shit-faced. I am drunk, but I thought I was handling myself skillfully until the pube comment.

"Well, the guys make less, that's for sure—like a few hundred a scene. The girls do better, up to one thousand or more depending on how well they're known and what they do."

"What they do?" Hilary asks.

"They make less for girl on girl, more for doing anal, gang bangs, things like that."

"I've never thought about it as a pay scale," Hilary says.

Since speaking isn't working out for me, I don't say how this system seems like incentive to do something you might not want to do, like, I don't know, a facial shot. I suppose we all do things we don't want to for money. I can never fully accept that people *choose* this profession because they simply adore screwing strangers on film. Or at least like it enough to justify the physical risks, emotional perils, and social stigmas.

Out of the corner of my eye, I see Simon rib Robbie and whisper something in his ear. They both laugh. I try to direct my attention to what Michel is saying, something about how the director of the porn shoot, Johnny Gun, used to be a porn star but is making the switch to directing. A few more guys have surrounded Robbie and are asking questions. I can't hear them. I feign interest in my conversation with Michel while I try to listen in. All I can discern are expletives like "dude," "no shit," and "crazy."

I excuse myself to go to the bathroom because I'm not fooling any-one with my toddler's attention span and my secret wish to cut Fedora

Girl for her pubic hair comment. I'm ready to go home. Once again, despite myself, I'm feeling uncomfortable and alienated. I want to take Robbie aside and ask what it was like, what it made him think and feel.

Instead, I confirm that my girly parts are, in fact, contained in my granny underwear, make a mental note to stop wearing them, and return to the kitchen where Robbie has thankfully lined up some kind of vodka shot. Mental escape is just what I'm looking for. We all throw one back, and Hilary and I head out to the balcony so she can smoke. I'm just drunk enough to smoke with her, and Canadian enough not to care about the so-called cold. We sit on folding chairs looking over the railing.

"Well, you're on bad behavior," she says. "Bad behavior," between us, is code for when I have no ability to control my facial expressions, which is often, but especially when they blatantly indicate that I don't like someone.

"That obvious?"

"Subtle as a flamethrower. But I get it. What was with that 'shaved' comment? She just wanted all those guys to think about her ponka."

"Totally. Did you see the way she hugged Robbie?" I say.

"No, I missed it, but he was practically boy-band swarmed in there."

"Do you go totally bare these days?" I ask.

"I have from time to time, but I still think the expectation that women shouldn't have pubic hair is preposterous. Not everyone is bare, by the way; we have to photoshop pubes off our AA models, or we just leave them. I think it's hot. So does my boss."

Hilary's boss is notorious for making crude comments, not to mention being in the news for sexual harassment lawsuits, so it's normal that she knows his preference in pubic hair.

"It's a lot of effort, right? Who has the time to *always* wax? And shaving is so fucking itchy! And immediately grows back!" I say.

"It's a nightmare. I'm always more excited to book a pedicure."

"What do you think, Hil? Do people in the porn business really love it or do it for the money?"

"I don't think it's many people's first choice. Maybe the men, but even then, it's kind of brutal."

"That's what I always think, but maybe we're just being judgmental."

"Probably," says Hilary. "I didn't attend that one semester of university not to feel self-important about some things," she jokes.

We stare out at the street, no closer to a conclusion about why people get into porn. Maybe one day I'll have the chance to ask them. We both butt out our cigarettes in an overflowing ashtray. Hilary says she's going to take off soon. She's meeting Tucker. I begin my attempt to corral Robbie. We are usually in sync with our desire to be the last ones at the party, for better or worse. But tonight, after power cleaning, and the party talk turning to cha-cha fashions, I'm done.

An hour later, after some sweet-talking, we are home tucked into our bed. As usual, as soon as Robbie's head hits the pillow, he begins to drift off.

"Thanks for taking me home," I say.

"No problem."

"Hey, what were all those guys talking to you about at the party?" I ask, running my fingers over his warm chest.

"What? Oh, mostly just making dirty jokes."

"Right, that's what I figured," I look around the dark room. Soon Robbie's breath turns into a snore. I count five helicopters whirl by. In the distance, police sirens howl. I roll on my side and try to tune out the noise. This, too, will take some getting used to.

Today I spent my day at home compiling transcripts from an inspiration-slaughtering focus group. In fact, I've been home typing out quotes from New Yorkers about their small-business American Express cards for the last two days, and I'm going postal. Why did I think I wanted to be a corporate writer again? The money, the visa—right, it was those convincing details. I probably could use a coworker, some banter over a coffee break, and a friend to meet for lunch. I only have one of those and she's busy. Today I was also, still, having a little trouble not thinking about the sex scenes Robbie's filming. But being domestic always helps me feel grounded—go figure—so midafternoon I hoofed it to the grocery store (with the double intention of getting out of my flying pig pajamas) and purchased ingredients for lasagna with homemade marinara sauce. Hours later, voilà—I'm dressed in adult clothes and have produced a bubbling, cheesy Pyrex. Go me.

We are eating my self-help lasagna while Robbie debriefs me on his day, which was another shoot with my new favorite producer, Nine. Apparently, his other contribution to the porn world, other than filming gonzo scenes with sketchy ethics, is mixing hip-hop and porn. What does that mean, exactly? Well, Robbie elucidates that it refers to making porn inspired by hip-hop or, conversely, watching porn to arouse the creation of beats. Either way, I'm still not sure I get it. Maybe I'm being small-minded.

This afternoon, Robbie attended a shoot with a DJ who was supposed to make a beat while two girls fooled around with each other. What that actually translated into was your regular old lesbian scene with a DJ watching.

"So hip-hop-meets-porn really just means substituting cheesy lounge music for rap?" I say.

"Yup."

"I guess you don't need a high-level concept in porn; it sells itself. What were the girls like?"

"Cute. One said she was doing porn to pay for her Masters' in Education."

"I bet that doesn't come up at parent-teacher conferences."

"The other didn't talk much about herself. But get this—she had a clit ring and it got stuck on the other girl's earring."

"No! That's awful!"

"Yeah, it put an end to things. She was in a lot of pain and had to ice it. She was really swollen."

"Ew."

"What? That's not gross. You get swollen when you're turned on. It's hot."

"I beg your pardon?" I say, pushing my plate away.

"Oh come on, you know you have bigger labia than some girls."

"I do?"

"Hey, that's not a bad thing!"

I cover my ears and stare at my husband-to-be. I am stunned. To be perfectly honest, I have never, not once in my nearly thirty years on the planet, considered the appearance of my labia. Frankly, I have rarely, if ever, even used the word, and I'm not that psyched to be using it now. Robbie can tell that he's thrown a boomerang and it's coming back his way.

"I love every little part of you," he says.

"Or big," I joke. "I know that, it's just . . . Wait, you've compared my labia to other girls you dated?"

"I guess I'm also thinking of what I see in porn, everything shows more when girls are totally bare."

"Keep digging."

We look at each other tentatively for a minute and sip our Zinfandel as if we're talking about who the next California governor might be, not labial folds.

"Like you've never compared my penis to other guys you've slept with," Robbie says. "Guys probably get judged in that department even more than girls."

"Fair."

"Can we let this go?"

"Yes," I say. "We can. Let's never discuss it again." I rise from the table and start cleaning up. His comment is so surprising to me that I'm actually without words.

"I have something else to talk about," Robbie says.

"Okay."

"Well, the assistant director that they hired on the show isn't working out and they're thinking of Matt. I wanted to know if you'd consider having him live with us if he takes the job. We can save some rent." Matt is our good friend from Montreal, and although I wasn't planning to live with another guy *and* my fiancé, the rent idea is compelling; our student-loan grace periods are almost up. As well, it might be nice to have someone else around while I'm settling into LA. I'm lonely.

"Okay," I say.

"Really?"

"Yup, two men and a porn show," I say. "Life is strange enough already. Bring it on."

The next evening, I'm changing into yoga clothes with Hilary at the Los Angeles Athletic Club when I ask, "Have you ever thought about the size of your labia?"

"Why no, not really," she says and laughs. She pulls a tank top over her head. "But you know who is super-self-conscious about hers is my friend Lindsay. She's mentioned it a few times. I think she's even considered getting them reduced."

"Reduced?"

"Yeah, labiaplasty. Lindsay told me a lot of porn stars do it. She's nuts about porn."

"Get out! They do not. Wait, Lindsay loves porn?"

"They do, and yes, I guess some women really dig it. Not me. All I need is my five-speed magic wand. It's so powerful you have to masturbate in jeans," she says. Her joke is lost on me since I'm earnestly thinking about my vagina.

"Maybe I need to step it up below the belt."

"You wouldn't get surgery, would you?"

"No, but maybe I should get a professional wax."

"There's a good esthetician here," she says, grabbing her yoga mat. "Shit, we're really late." We run up the stairs to class, taking them two at a time.

"Glad you could join us girls," our instructor, Dana, says as we enter the room and lay out our mats in the last spare inches. As I move straight into my first Downward Dog, Dana comes and presses the palm of his hand on my lower back. I feel like he can sense I need a little support, which is probably, as per usual, overthinking things, but I lean into his touch all the same.

"Focus on your breath," he says. "You have only three things to think about: your inhale, your exhale, and the space in between." I take in a deep sip of air and close my eyes in the position. Immediately, I feel calmer. My yoga practice has always been good for my sanity and self-esteem, which I realize has taken a few hits in the last little while. I have to remind myself that I'm going through a huge life change—moving, starting a new (boring and isolating) job, being engaged but keeping it secret from my closest friends, following my fiancé around—a guy who, incidentally, spends his day on porn sets—and now, the maraschino on top, considering a makeover for my cha cha. It's understandable that I'm not feeling totally Zen. I bet Siddhartha never stressed out about his pubic hair.

I'm thinking about things other than my breath, but my thoughts have slowed. With each warrior pose, I feel more in control, less like a snapped telephone wire. As we move into Tree pose, I stand in front of my reflection in the mirrored wall. Okay, so my labia (curse the word) are bigger than some other girls' labia. So what? I'm beautiful just the way I am! And gosh-darned Robbie loves me! Then I repeat the mantra, ignoring the urge to gag, and the critical voice telling me I sound like an *O Magazine* article.

By class's end, I decide that I will try a Brazilian wax. This is a new chapter in my self-exploration, the LA chapter. While I'm not signing up for labiaplasty, let alone a boob job just yet, or likely ever, barring breast cancer, I am curious what all the hype is about. Why do guys like the pubescent look so much? Have I judged it, shall we say, prematurely?

In Corpse pose I have an actual moment of silence. Just one. Broken when I realize how I need to convince myself that going bare was my idea before I could embrace it. In matters of sex, as in life, so much hinges on feeling in control. If Robbie had suggested I book a Brazilian the other day in bed, I would have smacked him. Hard. But I'm going to do it, and my main motivation is to be wanted by my man. Maybe that impulse can be empowering, if I let it. I want to be attractive to him, just as I wanted to be sexy for Trevor years ago. The desire to be desired is ever potent, as is, I suppose, my female competitive spirit. *Little does Robbie know he'll have*

Fedora Girl to partly thank for my new porn star look. It still annoys me that all men have to do is shower and get an occasional haircut, but I leave class feeling more accepting of the world as it is: totally fucked.

On my way out, I stop by the front desk to inquire about the wax. "She actually just had a cancellation," the receptionist says. "Do you want to take this slot?"

Five minutes later I am wrapped in a pale green robe, lying on a table, with a pretty Vietnamese woman inspecting my cha cha.

"Been a little while?" she says.

"Yeah," I exaggerate, *if a little while means forever.* To say that I feel exposed is an epic understatement. I feel like my grandmother just sent me a parcel containing the vibrator I accidentally left at her house over Christmas with a note that says: "Yours? I ran it through the dishwasher."

"How much do you want to leave here?" she asks, referring to my arboreal forest.

"Take it all off," I say, wishing that statement sounded more like it did at a bachelorette party I once attended. She nods and begins dumping baby powder all over my business, making me look not only hairy but also geriatric. I suddenly feel better about this makeover—get rid of that nasty old shit.

"Is the temperature okay?" she asks, as she smears on hot wax with a Popsicle stick and covers it with a strip of fabric.

"Yup," I say. Because I've done plenty of at-home waxing, I know this is the calm before the storm. The warm wax feels kind of cozy. The snap of a hundred hairs ripping out by the follicles that follows does not. Great, I only have to go through that, like, what, fifty more times?

"Okay?" she asks. I nod, since I am somewhere between wanting to scream and throw up.

"I'll get the worst part done first," she says and proceeds to remove the hair from where my landing strip would be if she were leaving one. She's right. It's the worst. I think I might fall off the bed if that's possible when you are lying securely on your back.

By the time she is fumbling around in my labial folds with tweezers I am so far beyond giving a shit, I'd need Doc Brown's DeLorean to get back there. On my way out, I give her a 50 percent tip because I figure that is the appropriate amount for someone who has just removed the hair from your ass crack.

Hilary is waiting for me in the lobby, frantically messaging her boss on her BlackBerry, as usual.

"So?"

"It's weird how evolving sexually means revisiting your ten-year-old genitals," I say.

"What's weirder is the article I recently read that says actual twelve-year-old girls are getting their bikini lines permanently laser-sculpted."

"You win," I say, and Hilary helps me hobble to the parking garage.

Last night I returned to an empty apartment. Robbie worked over-time, thanks to a highly unpunctual six-person gay shower scene, and then grabbed a late dinner with Michel. I was asleep by the time he returned, thus he hasn't yet made his pending baby-soft discovery. The sting has thankfully abated this morning. I arise before he wakes and run a bath where I froth myself into a vanilla-almond-scented lather. I've decided to reveal my Brazilian via a nonchalant naked entrance as I saw Jennifer Aniston do to get Vince Vaughn's attention in *The Break-Up*. Which is possibly the wrong cinematic inspiration. Whatever. I prop my feet up at the end of the tub and lady-razor my legs. I will take the visual approach. My man's a cinematographer and that's what this is about, after all. Seeing more. I emerge from the bath and towel off. Then I tie my wet hair in a topknot and don a white terry bathrobe. The morning is chilly, so in lieu of full nudity, I leave it untied and draped open. I peek downtown. Yup, there I am. I'm still not entirely sure how I feel about this stage four cha cha look. But here goes . . .

Or maybe I'll just make a quick coffee for us first. Who doesn't like coffee delivered to them in bed? I patter to the kitchen and fire up the espresso machine. Warm up milk. Tidy the dishes I neglected last night. Armed with two steaming cups, I return to the bedroom. Robbie is out cold, snoring with his mouth open, per usual. I place our mugs down on his bedside table and crack the blinds to let a few rays in. I let my robe fully part. He stirs, groaning and scratching his beard with his eyes still closed.

"Good morning," I say. "Coffee?"

"Mmm, hi," he mumbles sleepily. "What time is it?"

"Eight-thirty."

He grumbles again and cracks open his eyes.

"Here you are, my love," I say, handing him a mug. He takes a sip and then places it back down; his eyelids droop again. *Christ almighty, Robert.* "Notice anything different about your fiancée?" I probe, mildly annoyed at having to announce my reveal with a megaphone. *Perhaps first thing in the morning was not the best moment to get my man's attention.*

"What?" he peers at me again, scanning my face on down to my open robe. "Holy shit!" he exclaims as he registers my extra level of nakedness. He props up on his elbows. "Mmm, lovey, what's this about?" Now he's up.

"Just something new I'm trying," I say nonchalantly. "I figure if you can't beat 'em . . ."

"So hot," he says and pulls me toward him by my hips. He goes down on me. For a brief second I think: *Oh super, look how into me you are when I look like your porn star pals. A Brazilian wakes you up like a wailing fire bell.* Then I smack myself upside the figurative head. This was the point, Emily, duh. I focus on what's going on, which is good times. He slides my robe off my shoulders and pulls me onto the bed. The next ten minutes are a blur of hot sex: me straddling him as he moans admiringly at his new view. I finish first. Then we switch to doggie-style, his turn. Suddenly I'm into feeling like a hussy. I start to play the part a little. I turn around and say, "Ooh yeah, baby! More, baby!" He aims for my back, mostly landing mid-blades, except for the stream that whizzes past my shoulder and nails me in the earlobe. We both crack up.

"Sorry!" he says. I remain in the same position while he grabs a couple of tissues from the bedside table and hands me one.

"No problem," I say dabbing my ear. "Nice trajectory."

"Nice bare pussy," he says.

"Don't say 'pussy'!!" I yell.

"Seriously? If you're going to start acting like a porn star, you're going to have to get used to that word," he teases.

"Fine," I say as he wipes me up. I collapse on the bed. "Okay: pussy, pussy, pussy. Whatever. I hate that word. But I loved that."

"Me too," he says.

"So I get it."

"Get what?"

"It's like a freaking slip and slide down there. It's better than shaving. I get it. The porn stars are on to something on the friction front."

"Yup. *And* I like being able to see all of you."

"Jury's still out on that one for me, love muffin."

"You'll get used to it."

"Oh *will* I? Will *you* get used to your regular ball wax?"

"I'll do that for you. No problem. You should ask at your place if they do men. But I love you every which way, you know that." He leans in and kisses me where we now lie face-to-face on our respective sides of the bed. Content and sleepy again, we drift off for another hour.

I call Kate a little later, drinking my second coffee on the stoop.

"I got a Brazilian yesterday," I say.

"Oh yeah, I love my Montreal waxist," she says. "Like I would date her, if I liked girls. She's quick and painless. I think she's also actually Brazilian."

"Do you go bare all the time?" I say, surprised. *I guess you never know what your friends are up to in their underpants. Unless you regularly visit the steam room with them.* I watch several ants traveling the mini-grout highway between flagstones.

"Oh, hell yeah! I wear riding pants all day, every day. It's more hygienic."

"I don't know about *hygienic*. Isn't the purpose of pubic hair to give you a little barrier from the outside world? So that you don't get a trap-jaw ant up your cha cha or whatnot when you squat to pee in the Amazon?"

"Thanks for that image, Em. I don't live in the Amazon. I live in North America. I have a toilet."

"What about the growing-back-in phase? That's shitty, no?"

"It's not so bad. It gets better if you do it regularly. I barely have any hair on my legs from waxing religiously for years."

"Good for you. We'll see. I don't like being pressured into anything."

"You don't say."

We hang up and I go inside, sit down at my desk to get on with my workday. So Kate's on the Brazil train? Huh. Now I do see a few pros: like sensation and seduction factor, along with the obvious cons: pain, money, annoying patriarchal expectations. I guess I'll see how it goes. Or shall we say, how it *grows*. I take the last glug of coffee, prop one knee up, and open my PowerPoint doc.

CHAPTER 4

MILFS

"My period is late," I say to Kate over the phone.

"How late?"

"A few days—three or four, I think."

"Have you guys been careful?"

"As careful as usual; we're still using the pullout method," I say, as I push my shopping cart into the kitchen aisle at Target. I grab a poultry baster and toss it in.

"I can't believe you guys depend on that."

"That's what my gynecologist says. He calls it 'the pregnancy method.' But it's been working for four years."

"Well, take a test so you can stop worrying. Are you stressed? It could be stress."

"Yeah, I am. This move has been trying."

"Are you guys okay?"

"We are. Matt moved in yesterday. They're at some porn shoot in the Valley again today. I don't have any work to do this week, so I guess I'm feeling a little lost. I have no friends other than Hilary. Can you move here?"

"Maybe you should join a book club."

"Yeah, maybe, and perhaps I should pick up needlepoint as well. Do you own a meat thermometer?"

"Yes, it's essential for roasting a turkey. I have to get off my horse now," Kate says. "Call me when you take the pregnancy test."

I hang up the phone and continue my acquisition of kitchen essentials that Robbie neglected to acquire in his bachelorhood. What if I am pregnant? Crap, what if I'm pregnant in my wedding dress? What kind of dress suits a knocked-up bride? Empire waist, probably. Have we been acting completely naive and brazen with our birth control method after all? If I am pregnant, there's no question that we'll go through with it. We're engaged. We plan on starting a family *one day*. But it's not the plan right now.

I steer my shopping cart in the pharmacy direction. On my way, I pass the shoe department, the intimates, and the dreaded maternity wear. One glimpse of elastic-waist jeans conjures an image of my puffy-faced, varicose-veined self in tensor tights; I break into a jog. This cannot be. I stare, perplexed, at the broad selection of pink-lettered pregnancy tests. These fuckers are expensive. I grab a First Response and an EPT. This better not happen every month or I'll go broke. On my way to the end of the aisle, I grab a bottle of red nail polish and some exfoliating foot lotion. If I'm not pregnant, I will celebrate with a home pedicure. I heard once that you can't have pedicures when you're pregnant. I wonder if that's true. I know for sure I'll be giving up sushi, alcohol, unpasteurized cheese, and worst of all, my daily three espressos. Shoot me in the face.

Robbie and Matt now have an SUV to drive porn stars around in, which means that the Hyundai is mine to use. I pile my purchases in the trunk and make my way out of the maze of an underground parking garage. On my way through the exit, I stall twice, causing the old woman behind me to honk impatiently. I find this response not only abrasive but counterproductive. As an abominable driver, I'm always first to take the blame. But seriously, lady, would you like to start my car for me while I honk? On second thought, the old broad would probably be faster. *Ignore, relax, hold down clutch, turn ignition. Don't think about killing your hypothetical fetus in a car crash.* Two tries later, I'm off like a drunk in a golf cart.

Half an hour and several more pissed-off LA drivers later, I arrive back at the apartment. I am equally anxious to know my fate and desperate to avoid it, and with that in mind, I decide that Christina Ferrare's Lemon, Dijon-Roasted Chicken takes precedence. Besides, I don't have to pee. I pour myself a large Perrier and set to work rinsing and marinating a chicken.

My mother was twenty-eight, my age, when she had my older brother. My parents married at twenty-five and waited a few years before having kids. They waited longer than many of their peers. "We knew when the timing felt right," she's said to me before. I wonder if I will ever have that knowing feeling. Sometimes I like to imagine a hyperproductive version of myself with children. This Emily balances a baby on her hip while she blends organic baby puree. She nurses while penning a brilliant and moving novel. She balances home, career, and husband seamlessly. And she does it all clad in cashmere wrap sweaters, skinny jeans, and heels. Did I mention that this Emily looks a lot like Angelina Jolie? Suffice it to say, this Emily is fictional and the real Emily is much more likely to be contemplating sticking her head in an oven than to be selecting which

Jimmy Choos to wear to a playdate. She also seems much more concerned with herself than with her offspring. Wrong motivation. Crap.

While it's insanely unlikely that we'll ever be as financially prepared as the Jolie-Pitt clan, the truth is, we won't even be in as stable a position as our parents were at our age. Our combined student debt is nothing short of staggering. Our career prospects are tenuous at best. They say our generation—children of the baby boomers—will do less well financially than our parents. Historically, it's usually been the other way around. Oh well, who needs a house anyway? Any old roof will do. Medical insurance, on the other hand, seems pretty much a necessity for childbirth. I guess given the financial factors stacked against us, I can't expect to wake up one day feeling prepared for children. Ready to devote the .2 percent of myself that isn't obsessed with our own achievements and survival. My current sentiment is something more like panic with a dash of dread. Nonetheless, in my frenzy, I've prepared what promises to be a delectable roast chicken.

I am popping it in the oven when I hear the boys coming through the front door. I poke my head around the corner. As usual, the entryway is quickly cluttered with two sets of shoes and several black bags of film gear.

"Hey Emiloo," Matt calls, and Robbie walks over to give me a kiss.

"Hello, boys," I say.

"What are you making, my love?" Robbie asks. I crack the oven to show him and he grins. The three of us open Coronas and sit in the living room. I take a sip of mine and then set it down on the coffee table, realizing that this might not be the best moment for a cold one. Shit. I'm already bad at this. I meant to get this dang destiny-altering test over with before they returned. You can have an occasional beer when you're pregnant, right? The French don't give up wine and they still pop out snooty intellectuals willy-nilly. I'm one-fifth French Canadian. Well, then. I resolve to drink half.

"So, give me the details," I say. "What did you boys have the pleasure of filming today?"

"It was a Naughty American teacher-student scene with a porn star named Rylie Spence," Robbie says. "I guess she was big in the '90s?" He looks inquisitively toward Matt, who shrugs. "Anyway, she was bitching that she gets mostly MILF scenes now that she's older."

"How old is she?" I ask. Although I brought this topic up and do want to know the details, I can already feel myself becoming rigid. I take a slug of my beer. Maybe I'll drink three-quarters.

"Around thirty?" Robbie says.

"About that," Matt concurs. "But she looks older."

"Yeah, she does. She looks kind of haggard."

"So she's my age?"

"You're only twenty-eight."

"Twenty-nine in a month, that's around thirty."

"Okay, yeah, I guess. But she's probably lived pretty hard."

"Have you forgotten that I'd bartended for four years when you met me, dear? It's not exactly like I avoided nightlife." Robbie, wisely, doesn't bite and I tell myself to shut my trap. Nobody is making this age comparison but me, but I also feel defensive for Rylie. It sucks to have someone say you've "lived hard" without even knowing you. I guess that's the thing about being a porn star—you're going to be judged on various accounts.

"She produces and directs now, too," Robbie says, changing the topic. "Pretty hard-core stuff. Apparently she's trying to prove that woman directors can be just as raunchy, since female-directed stuff is known for being softer."

"Raunchy how?" I ask.

"Like fisting, choking, airtight scenes, that sort of thing."

"What's 'airtight'?" I inquire earnestly. Robbie darts a glance at Matt, who quickly looks down at his iPhone, avoiding eye contact.

"Well, it's," Robbie starts.

"I'm going to shower before dinner," Matt interrupts. He rises from the couch and swipes up his Corona from the coffee table.

"Okay, dinner should be another half hour or so," I say, looking up at him. He gives me a quick, awkward smile, says "K," and heads down the hall. I notice not for the first time that he's a pretty handsome guy, still retaining his college hockey player's physique; his dark hair and eyes contrast with soft, boyish features. Come to think of it, he has a bit of a Mark Ruffalo thing going on. I wonder if the "actresses" ever flirt with him. When he closes the bathroom door behind him, I look at Robbie. "Oops, I guess I scared him away," I say in a lowered voice.

"I don't think he's comfortable talking about this stuff around you. 'Airtight' is when a girl has a dick in her pussy, ass, and mouth at the same time—like that scene I told you about with the three black guys." Robbie suddenly changes the topic. "Hey, what was going on with you just there? You seemed like the age thing was upsetting you."

I wince as I think about that Valaria gonzo story I'd prefer to forget.

"Are you okay?" he asks.

"I don't know," I say. "The age thing is kind of crappy, don't you think? Men get older and all *George Clooney* and women get *haggard*."

"It's not like we're talking about all women. We're talking about porn stars. Youth is kind of a cache in this business. Most girls go into it at eighteen or nineteen and start getting cast as MILFs at twenty-three, that's what Rylie said. It's ridiculous, but it's not meant to be reality. Besides, I find older women hot. I'm with you, aren't I?" Robbie is a year-and-a-half younger than I and he is clearly joking.

I give him a deadpan stare. "Seriously though, I don't think I represent the average guy. In high school, I had a crush on a fifty-year-old teacher that nobody thought was attractive."

"So what you're saying is that you go for the older, ugly chick."

"Stop it!" he yells at me, smacking his Corona down on the coffee table. I jump at the sound. He leans back into the couch with an exasperated sigh. "I am not talking about *you.*"

I know that he isn't, and I know that I'm acting like I'm feeling insane. I don't know where to place all the various emotions that are running through me right now, which may or may not be the result of our discussion about aging and porn. I'm irritated, defensive, even a little mad. The double standards for men and women in this department are as annoying as they have always been—in porn, in Hollywood, and in life. What I should probably mention is the fact that my period is late and that the MILF discussion is hitting a little closer to home than usual, especially with the stubble barely growing back from my recent Brazilian. However, that confession would require me to open my mouth and actually say the words that I'm afraid of: *I could be pregnant.* If Matt would get out of the shower, then maybe I could just go find out. Instead I say, "So I couldn't even be a porn star if I wanted to anymore?"

"Come on, you could never have been a porn star," Robbie says.

"What?"

"Just talking about this stuff makes you uncomfortable! You think you could have sex, for money, on camera?"

"I don't know. Would you still have dated me if I were a porn star?"

"Sure."

"Really?"

"I might find it hard to know that you were off having sex with other people, but I think I could get over it."

"I don't think most guys would be okay with that scenario. I couldn't deal with you being a porn star."

"You don't say." He raises his eyebrows teasingly; his irritation softens a little.

We sit in silence for a minute, then he puts his hand on my knee and says, "I'm not most guys, Emily. Isn't that why you're marrying me?"

I stare at him, wanting to say so much, but then again, afraid of what I'm feeling in that moment: totally unsure of myself. What if I don't know this man (whom I could conceivably have a child with one day) so well, after all? Anyway, I'm sure he's being rhetorical. He's probably feeling defensive. Which annoys me, because the real message he's trying to send is, 'I can't believe you're calling me into question.' And he's right. Maybe I'm just pushing him to say something upsetting so that I can unleash all of the nebulous emotions I don't know how to express. I need to exit stage left before I start a major fight. I exhale, allowing my shoulders to drop two inches, and stand up.

"Do you want another beer?" I ask. He nods and I go to the kitchen to fetch him another Corona and check on my chicken. It's browning and bubbling gloriously, but the sight of it makes me furious. What am I doing roasting a goddamned chicken while my husband-to-be is off filming porn stars? Porn stars that he would apparently consider dating if I weren't around. Porn star being a profession he might earnestly consider. Are we too different to be signing up for a life together? Maybe Robbie is far too liberal for my tight ass. But I'm a mix of things, a smorgasbord of values—one thing is for sure, it's just like me to go about being all domestic and then resent the hell out of it. I open his beer and suffocate it with a plump wedge of lime.

"Here," I say, as I slap it on the coffee table.

"Gee, thanks," he says.

"You're welcome," I say, and then I unleash, despite my intention not to. "I hate all of these double standards! I hate the aging thing! Mostly I hate that you're perfectly fucking fine with all of this, and I'm this uptight prude! I bet the jackass in the porn industry who came up with the term *MILF* had *huge* mommy issues." I stand over him and punctuate my frantic gesticulations with a loud slap on my bare thighs. He looks up at me with his brow furrowed; he's dumbfounded by my outburst. I break eye contact with him and notice the evening light filtering through our dirty venetians. I can't wait to throw them in the dumpster.

"Do you want me to pretend to be uncomfortable?" Robbie says. "We've just had different exposure to this world. I don't think porn came up with MILF, by the way. Didn't you watch *American Pie*? That word went mainstream years ago. And if you think about it, MILF is actually a compliment. It's a really popular genre."

"No, I didn't watch that dumbass movie. I was busy backpacking in Peru with a Sylvia Plath book tucked under my hairy armpit," I say sarcastically. Except we both know it's the truth. Our formative years were different. He ate Big Macs and enjoyed blockbuster teenage comedies. I eschewed meat for tempeh and exclusively watched Lars von Trier.

"Right." Robbie looks utterly defeated.

"My period is late."

Robbie goes white. "What? Is *that* what this is about?"

"Sort of. I don't know. Not totally." I wither onto the blue IKEA armchair on the other side of the coffee table from him. I stare at my toes in red flip-flops; they still badly need that home pedicure they may or may not get.

"How late?"

"Three or four days. I have a test. I meant to take it before you guys came home but I was busy being Martha Stewart."

"When did you realize this?"

"Today, shopping at Target." And then I suddenly blurt out, "I don't think I want to have a child."

"*Ever?*" says Robbie, looking increasingly aghast.

"I don't know, not now." I move over to the couch and sit next to him, push my shoulder against his, and look down at my fingernails, gnawed to the quick. They, too, need serious TLC.

"Yeah, it's not the best timing," he admits. We look at each other and I feel myself well up. My propensity to cry mid-conversation, let alone at the prompting of nostalgic car commercials, is well-known to Robbie. He grabs my hand but doesn't question my tears.

"This is all, just . . . a lot," I blubber. At that moment, Matt slinks out of the bathroom with his head and waist wrapped in towels, à la Ferris Buehler. We lock eyes for an instant and he gives me a "sorry for existing" smile, then he shuffles quickly down the hall. *Goof.* He shuts the door to his room, now dubbed "the Man Cave" because of how often he disappears in there for five-hour stints with the blinds closed. I look back at Robbie.

"I know it is. You'll take the test and then we'll know. We'll deal with whatever. You'd be a yummy mummy, by the way." He gives me a sly grin and nudges my shoulder back with his. I squeeze his hand in return.

"Thanks, but not a good one. I just drank a beer," I sniff, sucking back snot.

"That's okay."

"Why does talking about all of this upset me so much?"

"Porn or pregnancy?"

"Porn. Duh," I say with a little laugh, and wipe my nose with the back of my hand.

"Do you think maybe it would be better not to discuss it?"

"No, I want to know what you do all day; I want to know what you think about it. I just wish it didn't bring up so many feelings. It bothers me that women are lumped into these narrow stereotypes—how can you go from barely legal to MILF in three years? Thirty is like sixty-fuck-ing-five in porn years."

"I didn't write the rulebook."

"I know, but who did? I hate that asshole! And I detest that no mat-ter how dumb I think these standards are, there's still a part of me that wants to fit into them. You know? But I don't even know whether that means I do, or *don't,* want to be a MILF! It's so confusing!" My hands fly up through the air again. From outside it must look like I'm doing the wave, but faster, angrier.

Robbie, calm in the way a parent becomes when they realize their frustrated child just needs to vent, smiles and says, "Let's just get this test over with. Can we? I think we're muddling the issues."

"Okay, yeah." I let Robbie give me a hand up from the couch and lead me into the bathroom, which is comfortably steamy. God, I would so much rather be standing under a hot shower right now instead of squat-ting over the toilet. He sits on the edge of the bathtub while I pee on the dipstick, which he takes from me unflinchingly when I finish. We sit in silence and wait for the timer on his phone to beep.

The test, he informs me, is negative.

There are few professions that demand as much perfection of a woman's body than that of a porn star. Model, perhaps, then actress, then retail sales girl at, say, Abercrombie and Finch or Forever 21, where I swear they must not sell anything over a size four. I won't harp on this for too long, because while I don't know a single woman who doesn't have a delusional body image, I don't blame the porn world per se. I don't pin it on anything or anyone, actually. I have to live in the world, and I prefer to do so without being angry. We girls have to stay high-minded to filter out the many negative messages out there. But speaking briefly of messages, here are a few zingers that I've heard in the past few years:

One: Howard Stern iterated that the perfect height and weight for a woman was five-foot-nine, and 110 pounds. Yup, you heard me, five-foot-nine, 110. Unsurprisingly, he was referring to a porn star's height and weight when he uttered that nugget of wisdom. Howard just loves porn stars. Good for him! I'm five-foot-two-and-a-half and I weigh more than that. What a fuckwad.

Two: A forty-one-year-old male acquaintance of mine had the audacity to say, "Twenty-three is the perfect age for a girl because her body is still hot, but she has no expectations." Side note that made me feel better: His twenty-three-year-old girlfriend dumped him shortly after that. Loser! Side note to make him feel better: He was promptly invited to a Halloween party at the Playboy mansion, where he immediately recovered. Damn.

Three: A totally smart, affable guy friend let fly this: "Every woman would be hotter with a boob job."

"No, not you too!" I said. I had a boss at the time who shared his opinion. He suggested I'd be way more attractive with D-cups. I believe his actual words were, "A few cup sizes could bring you up to an eight." What was I starting at, douchebag? Four? I didn't quit, at least not for that comment. I resigned when after a charity event he tried to grope me, wouldn't take no for an answer, and I had to throw myself out of a moving limo.

While I often take the stance that dumbass comments are best ignored, these statements are obviously lodged in my psyche somewhere, along with my constant desire to lose five to ten vanity pounds. Lucky for my significant other, it's only in my primary relationship that I have hissy fits about MILFs.

I don't know whether to consider MILF an insult or a compliment. Is "mother" a little pejorative because it suggests being past your prime? And is middle age, in a sexual context, always construed as a little desperate, a little *Real Housewives of Wherever*? In some ways, *MILF* doesn't seem like a very powerful term for women. Think about it: whether you're a Mother He'd Like to Fuck, as opposed to a Mother He Would Not Like to Schtup, is ultimately up to him.

Then again, if you flip it around so that a MILF is a seductress, a temptation-wielding force, then everything changes. Controlling men's desire can be quite powerful, after all; just ask Shakespeare. I've heard several porn stars say that they like the sense of power they get from doing XXX—inspiring hundreds of thousands of men to get off on them. I can see that. In this interpretation, *MILF* clearly equals compliment. He wants *me*—*this* hot mama—bad. Besides that, there are plenty of examples to prove that older, powerful women are sexy—Demi Moore, Courtney Cox, Helen Mirren for the Baby Boomers. It can be argued, in our stunted-adulthood society, that youth is no longer the hot commodity it once was. According to Sugar DVD—a Netflix-type porn service—MILF is one of the most popular porn genres—second only to interracial (which apparently is pretty popular). And on Youporn.com, it is among the top ten most searched. Barely legal is out, cougars are in. Go team!

Where I've ultimately landed on the insult-versus-compliment issue is somewhere in the vicinity of not caring. Who has the time to think about whether she's old or young, hot or not, in whoever's damn opinion? One just has to eat her leafy greens or eschew them for chocolate-covered donuts, decide whether to spring for the boobs or the Botox, and focus on other things. Of course, we all know that's easier said than done, with access to the worst invention ever for a woman's body image: the Internet. As I write this, it is noon, I haven't left the house, and I've already seen five ads for how to melt belly fat. I briefly clicked on one—the nonsense about a Brazilian fruit that magically counters cheese fondue.

Alas, if I knew then what I know now, I'd have an easier time taking it all less personally. Maybe we get less self-centered as we age, or perhaps just happier to get any ego bolstering at all. Either way, time struts on in her uncomfortable stilettos.

For the moment, Robbie and I are lying in bed on a lazy Sunday with hazy sunshine filtering through the blinds. Birds are chirping outside, which makes me wish I liked chirping birds. We have been waking and drifting back off for the last hour—my very favorite way to rise. It's been a couple of days since the pregnancy scare. I am thinking about various ways to pass the day. A trip to the Fairfax Flea Market to buy some refurbished furniture? Perhaps we can think about the wedding guest list that we've been meaning to get around to. It's a doozy, thanks to Robbie's two million cousins. On second thought, maybe just brunch followed by an afternoon matinee at The Grove is the ticket. Of course, we still need to tell our friends and family and set a date. First things first. Robbie spoons me from behind, stretching his arm across my side and reaching up to grab my boob.

"Well hello there," I say.

"I was just having a sexy dream about you," he says.

"Mmm, that's fun. What about?"

"We were in your old Vancouver apartment. You were straddling me, and I had you pinned in the doorway," he says.

"Yummy."

"And then I flipped you around and started doing you in the bum."

"Keep dreaming," I say.

"Sure you don't want to try?" he asks.

"Not unless you have a hefty supply of morphine."

"It doesn't have to be painful," he says.

"Who told you that? One of your porn-star friends?"

"Seriously, you just have to warm up. Those girls sit on a dildo for half an hour before they start a scene."

I turn around and look into my husband-to-be's watery blue eyes. Sleepy crow's feet creep to his hairline, making him look older and wise. As usual, he is wearing just a t-shirt in bed, a pale pink one at the moment. His beard is sporting a dollop of morning drool—he's a mouth breather due to a deviated septum and an unfortunate condition called "non-allergenic rhinitis." I love this man enough to find all of these details completely adorable. Love is weird like that. But if he thinks this blissful Sunday is kicking off with a dildo in my ass, boy is he wrong.

"So that's a no?" he says.

I flip off the warm comforter, sigh, and push myself up out of bed.

CHAPTER 5

ANAL

I'm sitting on our flagstone steps, waiting for Robbie to pull up. Even though it's past six, the summer sun is still bright and high, and it feels good on my exposed décolletage. I peer down my shift dress at my beige strapless bra—do we call it décolletage with A-cups? Anyway, I'm rocking my closest equivalent to cleavage. I second-guess my navy silk frock and strappy heels, wondering if Robbie will find it a bit dressy. Then again, he's surrounded by nude women all day, most of them covered in nothing but bodily fluids by shoot's end. A classy dress is probably refreshing—even sexy—by comparison. We're headed to Fridays Off the 405, a night of live music at the Getty Museum. I've been anticipating this all day. I love the Getty—it's free, full of art, and its sprawling symmetry is more soothing than a piña colada. I could lie on the sun-warmed tiles for hours listing to trickling fountains and staring at passing clouds, if only security guards wouldn't ask me if I was having a medical emergency. Robbie pulls up and I hop in the Hyundai. He's dressed in work attire: black cargo shorts, a bright orange t-shirt, and Pumas. There are no suits in the reality TV biz. He's underdressed; I'm overdressed. But it works. We exchange a quick kiss, and then he peels down the street in his usual getaway manner.

"I spoke with your mom this afternoon," I say.

"Nice, how is she?"

"She's great! She wanted to know how long we're staying with them in the country. I said I thought it was Thursday to Monday." Robbie and I are planning a trip home in two weeks for a dose of Canadian summer and to finally announce our engagement. First, we'll stop to see my family in Halifax, where Robbie will oh-so-formally ask my father for my hand in marriage. Then we'll continue on to Montreal to see his two sets of parents. Both Robbie's mom and dad have country houses in the same Laurentian lake region, so we'll lake-bounce. Not the worst way to pass time. Not the easiest to organize.

"Monday? I thought we agreed we'd move to my dad's on Sunday morning and give him the second half of the weekend. He always gets the shaft on weekends." Robbie merges onto the 101 and into the far left lane in the same amount of time it would have taken me to check my blind spot. I white-knuckle the door handle as if it's liable to fly open, rip off, and leave me flailing to execute a James Bond move.

"Oh, I didn't remember that. I said it all tentatively."

"Yeah, but now she's going to be disappointed when I tell her we're going to Dad's on Sunday morning. Great."

"Sorry, she sounded really excited to see us. I guess I wanted to go with the momentum." When Robbie's mom gets pumped about plans, which is often, you feel left out if you don't start climbing decibels along with her—the conversational equivalent to swinging from the rafters. I don't like to let anyone imbibe or swing from metaphorical rafters alone.

"I know, but now I have to put a negative spin on the weekend already."

"She'll understand, babe," I say, and put my hand on his over the gearshift.

"She'll understand but that doesn't mean she'll be happy." He sounds mildly annoyed by my gaff. Oops.

"Well, maybe we should cut out Wednesday night in the city with our friends and stay at her place four nights; that would help."

"But you wanted to see your girlfriends in Montreal that night, luv," he says more gently, reminding me that this will require rearranging my plans with friends to better suit family. It's not the first time we've dealt with this dynamic. It likely won't be the last. It's nice of him to double-check, but I'm genuinely feeling accommodating.

"I know, but maybe I can convince them to come meet me in the country for lunch or something."

"Are you sure?" he probes. Translation: *You're saying yes now but are you going to be annoyed later?* He's been to that town and knows it's no fun.

"Yeah, for sure. I'll see if it can work."

"You're the best," he says, and appreciatively squeezes my silk-covered upper thigh. I fiddle with the radio and land on 93.5 Back in the Day Hits, and Young MC is rapping like it's 1989. Robbie sings along. Planning our summer vacation has made me slightly anxious. Even more anxious than the 80 miles per hour he's currently driving. It's not just because we have mammoth news—"Heya, how are things? I'll be the mother of your grandchildren! *If* we have them! Hope you like me!"—but also because the in-law time-share is clearly something I'm still getting used to. I should have kept my damn mouth shut. Divorced parent expectations are not my forte, since they are not my personal, nuclear experience. Sure, while both his parents have long since found other partners and are happy, they nonetheless covet their time with their child, especially when they have to split their vacations and holidays in half with him. When you factor in that Robbie doesn't like conflict or disappointing people, it's a match made in WASP-guilt heaven—which is just like Catholic guilt, only with more innuendo and gin.

After a relatively brief twenty-minute hiatus in gridlock, we merge onto the 405. Soon I can see the Getty Center perched on the sunburnt hills in the distance. It doesn't look like more than slabs of concrete from here, but Richard Meier knew what he was doing with the stuff. Each square that forms the center is thirty inches, or a ratio thereof. I don't know shit about geometry, but the resulting effect is sublime. From the west-facing terraces, the Pacific stretches all the way to Asia. Surrounded by all that sun-warmed sediment, all that art, you expect a Greek tragedy to unfold. It's time to forget about niggling travel plans. We pull into the parking lot, where the Getty Center makes up for the free art—fifteen-dollar parking. The parking garage is enormous, but it's already just about full. We snake down to the bottom level, somewhere I never hope to be in an earthquake, and ride the elevators up to the tramway. The line to board is long but moving steadily. Robbie and I join in and stand holding hands among the crowd of twentysomethings. We appear to be some of the older people in the crowd. These days, I like the feeling. Being engaged makes me feel slightly superior to my former self. This self knows where she is going, what she wants. Today's Emily manages in-law expectations and roasts chickens for dinner; yesterday's Emily shook six martinis at a time and always saw the lights come on at last call.

"So?" I say.

"So?" Robbie and I have existed in silence for the better part of the last hour, save for the odd perfunctory comment. We often do this. I was struck by Robbie's aversion to lame small talk and gossip immediately when we started dating. I liked that about him. While I'm not exactly Chatty Cathy myself, I'm still usually the first one to break the silence. My disinclination toward small talk butts up against my fear of becoming married people with nothing to say. At the moment, small talk wins.

"What happened in your day?" I ask, unconvinced I really want to know the details, but curious nonetheless.

"Not too much actually, it was pretty mellow," he says.

"What were you filming?" Each day I tell myself I won't probe. I won't ask things like "Where have you been? What have you been watching? Is there a faint odor of sex on your person or am I imagining things?" But every damn day I ask anyway. I don't believe this bodes well for my grown-up powers of wifely self-restraint. Perhaps I still have a ways to go.

"Well, the plan was to film two guys doing anal with this girl at some Sherman Oaks mansion but the girl couldn't take it."

"Take it?"

"Yeah, literally. I heard her telling the director that she'd done such a rough anal scene the day before, that she was too sore. She had to stop."

I notice a pixie girl with an ironic tiger on her t-shirt dart us a look as she slides before us onto the tram. Robbie and I cram into a corner and hold the handrail. "I don't know how anyone can get fucked like that," I whisper.

"It's all about proper warm-up," Robbie says. "I told you the other day—they sit on dildos for half an hour while they do their makeup."

"Oh right, I forgot that charming detail. Now *they* can think about it too." I gesture to the couple seated below us who are oblivious to our conversation, intensely petting and staring into each other's eyes. We both laugh. I stare at their private oblivion for a moment longer. We used to be like them. Robbie snaps me out of it.

"I don't understand," he says with a sly grin. "You liked it that first time."

"Oh Christ, I was really hungover."

"Maybe I should get you drunk tonight."

"Done. But you're still going to have to accept that I don't have a natural aptitude in this department. It's not like I'm so closed-minded that I've never tried. It's just painful for me, even with so-called proper warm-up. I think porn is misleading, they make it look too easy."

"You hold a lot of tension there. You need to relax."

"Thanks, that's really relaxing." I roll my eyes and look out the window. "You know, I think maybe you have some Freudian anal fixations. How come all women suddenly have to be willing to go there just because guys watch it in porn constantly? Doesn't that girl today prove that maybe we're not all built for that type of rigorous backdoor action?" We make our way up the long staircase, following the crowd and the sound of music in the distance. We walk through the central rotunda building and outside again into the main open-air terrace.

"Not all guys like anal. But anyway, people were into it long before porn," Robbie says. We both stop and survey the scene—a stage is set up and a large crowd surrounds it. On the periphery, vendors sell beer and wine.

"Sure, in ancient Greece. But it's way more popular in the mainstream than it used to be twenty years ago. Don't you remember that conversation we had with your dad once—about how in his day it was hard to convince a girl to give you a blowjob? Now you're a prude if you don't take it in the rear like a pro."

"When did we talk about blowjobs with my dad?"

"I don't know, some after-dinner port-fueled conversation. He probably didn't word it like that. Don't you think you're more into anal because you've watched porn all your life?"

"Probably."

We join a line for the concession stand. It's time for a beverage to go with this conversation.

"Porn gets so repetitive that they just have to keep penetrating different holes to make a whole film," I say. "Cha cha, ass, eyes, ears . . ."

"Some women like anal more than you do. Rylie Spence says it's her favorite sexual position. It gives her the most intense orgasms. What do you want to drink?"

"That's such bullshit," I scoff.

"Okay. What should I order you?"

"She's just saying that because she wants to fulfill a male fantasy— yours, apparently," I hiss. "I know some girls like it more than I do, but no girl loves getting rammed in her exodus apparatus by several guys for hours at a time. I'll have what you're having."

"I've met some recently who do," he says matter-of-factly, and joins the line of concertgoers to order. I move away from the hipster fray to the railing overlooking the manicured gardens. It looks peaceful down there, perfect, surreal. I want to dive into it. I close my eyes and imagine the fall. Robbie comes up behind me and hands me a tall plastic cup of beer. "Why are you being so defensive?"

I sigh and take a swig of cold ale. Certainly he's asking the right question. Why am I? One crass and honest reason is that I don't like my fiancé comparing my asshole with other girls' assholes and their gaping abilities. But I don't say that. I'm also afraid that I'm fast becoming the vanilla sex girl compared to what he sees at work. We're not new anymore. We haven't had explosive sex in a semipublic place for, what, a year? Now we're walking the path to matrimonial bliss, otherwise known to some as the death march of sexual attraction. I know that's not my burden to shoulder exclusively. Keep sex exciting! Be eternally hot! (Or cute and sexy or whatever version of that I am.) Be enough to sustain his insatiable male libido FORVER! A politician's wife I met at a party once told me: "Have sex whenever he wants to. That's how you keep a marriage together." I almost spit out my tepid Chardonnay when she said it. Then I walked away wondering if it's kind of true. Does that also include *however* he wants to? Too bad I can't go back and ask her. Should I tell Robbie that my criticisms of ass sex are perhaps rooted in a fear of abandonment? That if I don't satisfy him, he will cheat or leave me? That I sometimes feel pushed to be a certain way sexually for all the wrong motivations, and may well end up resenting the hell out of it? Of him? How dare he put me in this corner and force me to have anal or be sexually uninteresting, forgettable, alone.

"Em?"

"What? I'm fine, I'm just thinking."

"I see that."

"I guess it feels like a lot of pressure to be up for anything all the time, like a porn star."

"Hey, that's not my intention. I *am* aware that it's a profession." My hair, twisted in a messy bun, is coming undone and spinning in the wind. He gently tucks a few pieces behind my ear.

"I know." I feel myself soften. Of course it's not his objective to make me feel all of these things. He doesn't even know that I feel them, and I don't know where to begin to explain. "Let's go check out the music." I hold out my hand and he takes it in his always warm palm. We walk away from the railing, the darkening sky, and into the crowd, which is swaying to amorphous indie rock. Ironic facial hair, skinny jeans, and lanky-framed women in vintage peasant dresses abound. They all wear impassive expressions. I suddenly feel desperately uncool. I'm better dressed for the ballet. I feel alone, out of touch, as if no one here could possibly have my dumbass sex issues.

Admittedly, I did a little research on the subject of anal sex. Turns out, according to a study by the *Journal of Sexual Medicine*, that young women are much more interested in backdoor action than ever before. In fact, 40 percent of women from the ages of twenty to twenty-four say they've tried it. Why the sudden spike in anal sex among the younger set? Are they just more open to discussing it? Genuinely interested? Or both?

Hmm. Considering that the popularity of anal sex has increased alongside the growing consumption of Internet porn, it suggests there's a monkey-see-monkey-do kind of thing happening here. It's no wonder, when a quick glance at mainstream porn would have us believe that most women thoroughly enjoy anal sex instigated with little to no foreplay, and that we gals orgasm willy-nilly from this act alone. Suffice it to say, anal sex occurs online with greater frequency, ease, and lack of communication than it does in real life. Real life is messy, nuanced. And most girls I know aren't always freshly waxed, anally bleached, and in the mood. It isn't a bad thing that porn is encouraging us to spread our horizons, if you will. What's important is that we're communicating about this phenomenon rather than acting out of perceived porn-spawned expectations. So are we?

The study mentioned above suggests that many women are. Ninety-four percent of women who reported having anal sex in their last encounter also had an orgasm. Damn! Is anal sex better for orgasms than a five-speed magic wand? The rationale, as interpreted in William Saletan's *Slate* article "The Ass Man Cometh," is positive. It seems that the more sexual acts a woman is engaging in, the more likely she is to orgasm. And anal sex often happens in tandem with other sex acts— vaginal, oral, and partner masturbation. Saletan explains: "Women who were getting what they wanted were more likely to indulge their partners' wishes. It wasn't the anal sex that caused the orgasms. It was the orgasms that caused the anal sex."

More guys initiate anal sex, which girls engage in as part of a give-and-take. *Okay, sure, that sounds familiar.* The attitude of mutually giving and receiving can create a willing space to explore new things. From porn-inspired fantasies to the bedroom, seamlessly—win-win.

In a recent *Elle* magazine article called "The Imposter," Tracy Clark Flory tells a different story about how Internet porn affected her sex life. She revealed that although she's been a regular sex columnist and sex-positive advocate for years, up until recently she faked her orgasms. She had lots of sex, good sex, but she had difficulty being orgasmically honest with her partners—i.e., explaining that it would take X + Y + Z to get her there. Instead, she put on repeat Broadway performances to maintain an illusion of who she thought she should be in bed. She learned many of these presumed male expectations from porn. She says: "I had strong feminist political inclinations, but I was also deeply afraid of male rejection . . . What if I didn't orgasm and was labeled as frigid or repressed? . . . Internet porn had taught me that sexy, desirable women orgasm at the drop of a thong, and I wanted to be a temptress—aggressive, insatiable, and uninhibited."

I see my former self clearly in this description. That night, stewing in my emotions at the Getty Center, I both resented the expectation that I was supposed to have sex like a porn star and desperately wanted to live up to the fantasies he encountered each day at work. Instead of seeing this fictitious world as something separate or even complementary to our sex life, I compared myself with it and felt that I came up short. How dare he bestow such a burden upon me?

Except, oops, he didn't. I did. In an attempt to please everybody, I often exaggerated and internalized expectations, sexual and otherwise, in a way that left me ultimately defiant and resentful. Tracy eventually found a way out of her pattern by communicating genuinely with a guy she loved and trusted. A fairy-tale ending, of sorts.

Alas, like most things in life, sometimes things are easier comprehended in retrospect than done.

At eight the next morning, I wake fuzzy-headed from the Getty Center tap beer. Robbie is still comatose, so I leave him in bed and slink to the kitchen to make coffee. It's a sunny July day in Southern California, per usual. I spoon espresso into our stovetop maker and warm up some almond milk. I've never liked regular milk, and my mom never pushed it, much to the chagrin of a soccer mom who once tried to make me drink it at her dinner table. I called my mom and told her I was being held under duress. She immediately sped over in our silver Chevy station wagon and scooped me up. *Hmm, maybe it's such childhood treatment that still has me believing I'm a special flower.* As the espresso maker begins to bubble, my phone rings. It's my girlfriend Kate, calling from Canada with the benefit of three hours ahead.

"Good morning," I yawn.

"Hi!!! Is it obnoxiously early to call on a Saturday?"

"Yes, and that greeting is even more pleasant with a hangover, but I'm up."

"Good, I'm driving to the barn and I wanted company. What did you do last night?"

"Went to see some live music at the Getty Museum with Robbie, discussed anal sex, drank beer."

"That's pretty, minus the middle part."

"What are your thoughts on the matter?"

"Oh, I don't know, I tried it with Mark." Mark was Kate's longest boyfriend, clocking in at five years.

"Did you like it?"

"Sure, to a point. I think it has to be with someone you really trust. And more importantly, someone not too girthy." She pauses. I can hear the wind from her open car window. "I guess you could say it's on the menu, but I don't order it every day of the week."

"Right, I wouldn't even say it's on the standard menu in our house. It's more like a seasonal feature. This analogy is kind of gross."

"When are you getting here already?"

"Two weeks!"

"Amazing, I've already started planning your welcome dinner. We'll do it outside on the patio—wine, tapas, sound good?"

"About that . . ."

"No."

"There's been a bit of a conflict."

"No!!"

"Yeah, I screwed up the dates when I was talking to Rob's mom. You know me, I never even know what month it is. Now I think we have to spend an extra night in the country. Any chance you can come up there?"

"No way! I want to see *you*, not Robbie's whole family." I pour my coffee and take it out onto the front stoop. She continues, "Sorry, but you know what I mean. Ever since you started dating Robbie, me and Steph barely get to see you. It's bad enough you moved away, but every time you come back to Montreal we have to fight to get a night in. Doesn't his family know you had a whole life here before them? We were your family first."

"I gather you and Steph have discussed this."

"Well, it's fucking annoying!"

"It's really not their fault. I screwed up the dates. I'll just tell Robbie that we can't go to the country on Wednesday, okay?"

"Good."

"My head hurts, I have to not speak."

"Fine, I'll call someone else."

Kate hangs up. I know she's not really mad at me; she's just in one of her bulldozer moods. I love that she always tells me exactly what she thinks and never minces words, but she's not exactly what you'd call mild-mannered. Honestly, if it's a question of disappointing Lynn or Kate, I don't really know whom I'm more afraid of. Just wait until I tell Kate that Robbie's clan will be my actual family, legally.

An hour later, I'm lounging on the couch with a magazine when Robbie appears in the doorway in a shirt and nothing else. He absently pulls it down, which does nothing to hide his patently naked bottom half.

"Hi cutie," I say.

"Why aren't you in bed with me?" he mumbles.

"Couldn't sleep."

"Come back."

We climb back into bed together and Robbie initiates a cuddle maneuver that to me is more *water torture* than *expression of love*.

"Ten seconds," I say, referring to how long I can stand to have his tree-trunk legs and arms draped over me, redirecting my blood supply.

"No!" he moans as I heave his thigh off my midsection. I roll onto my side and he sidles in warm behind me. "Are you hangover horny?" he teases. His midsection pushes into my derrière. I know where he wants this to go.

"What? Oh, *that*. I don't know." My headache has faded and I am in that sleepy yet buzzy postbooze haze, well-known to me, where I lie thinking about the million things I could accomplish today but lack the real enthusiasm to execute them. Is anal sex one of those tasks? Surely it shouldn't be a task in the first place. It should spring from my natural desire, right? I think it did once. Or at least it should originate from my inclination to please Robbie. I have that chip—the giving one; I know I do. Where did I stash it? Why is being asked and/or probed by half-asleep, spooning fiancé such a weighty buzzkill these days?

The same way ping-ponging between what my mother-in-law-to-be wants from us and what Kate wants from me makes me not want to do any of it. Piss off, everyone! I'll stay home, set up a hammock on the lawn, and read a book. Voilà—a vacation for one. Want me to be a sex goddess? I'll be a nun. Take that! Alas, I'm a little too late for the monastery.

I turn and kiss Robbie because I have enough sense to know that I'm not my best self these days and that making out is a better aphrodisiac than overthinking. Robbie reaches one hand to my cheek—a move he knows makes me melt, and proceeds to kiss my neck. He looks me in the eyes and I remember that this is him and me, not a script. There are no absolute dos and don'ts. I love this man.

"Maybe just the tip? I'll make it worth your while," he whispers with a twinkle in his eyes. I crack up.

"Perhaps," I say, rolling on top of him. True to form, a bit of kissing gets me going. Turned-on, I'm now feeling magnanimous and more adventurous. "Okay, you win. Let's try again."

"Seriously?" Robbie says. He lights up like a boy ripping the Christmas wrapping off his favorite video game.

"Yup, you get the lube."

Twenty minutes and plenty of awkward maneuvering later, the deed is done. Or, *er*, wholeheartedly attempted. As usual, I spent a good portion of the event trying to think about soothing things like the ocean at sunset but wound up picturing scenes from *Braveheart*. Meanwhile, I barked instructions like a volleyball coach: "To the left! Wait for it!" Sometimes it helps when he just holds still for a second while I breathe deeply. But a second turned into two minutes, which of course led to a semi-erection and we had to start all over again. Lucky me.

"I bet you didn't think I would take you literally when you said, 'Just the tip,'" I joke, lying next to him now and twisting my tangle of tousled hair into a knot.

"But the tip is the worst part," Robbie says matter-of-factly, splayed postcoital with one arm behind his head. "Once you have the tip in, it gets easier."

"But it goes against all my instincts!" I say. "My impulse is: Ouch! Get that fucker out of there!"

"Well then we need to work you up to it more," he says earnestly. "It's not like all porn stars were just born with this natural ability. It takes practice."

"Oh, here we go. I should sit on a dildo while I transcribe focus groups. I know, I know." I stretch my legs up into the air and grab my ankles in a deep stretch. It feels great.

"No, seriously," he turns toward me and props up on one elbow. "There's a reason it's so painful—I think you hold a lot of your stress there. You like it when I massage your butt, right?"

"Mmm hmm," I concur.

"Well you need to think of anal sex as the pinnacle point of an awesome deep-tissue massage. What we need is a three-month game plan." He sits up fully. My ass is now in his face; my toes graze the wall behind us in what's known in yoga as Plow position. "The first month is exclusively massage, then we move on to small toys, and eventually work up to the real deal." I laugh. Robbie doesn't. His blue-grey eyes are court-defense serious. "I think it could really help you," he continues, "with your occasional insomnia, constipation, all of it!"

"You did not just suggest ass sex as a remedy for my constipation! And how do you know that?" I maneuver back down and shimmy under the top sheet.

"Oh please, we're getting married, Emily. I've seen you with your Bran Buds and Benefiber," he says. "It's all linked to tension, right?"

"Yeah, I guess, and hydration. Who are you? Dr Oz? The ass-sex yogi?"

"Just someone with your best interests at heart." He leans over and kisses me softly.

"And yours," I tease, except it's the thinly veiled truth. I'm pushing my boundaries for him. At the moment, I'm okay with that. It strikes me as cute that he's trying to convince me that there are unseen side benefits for me in this. He doesn't seriously expect me to get on a three-month plan to having ass sex like a porn star, does he? *The first month sounds nice. Maybe I'll just call ollie-ollie-oxen-free after that.* I shake my head. How did I manage to find the least squeamish man on the planet?

"Thanks for having my back, handsome," I tease. "But I am *not* about to get on any butt-sex plan. I'm still trying to finesse my find-a-job plan." I give him a sly grin and reach over and kiss him. "But maybe we can try again sometime soon . . ." I toss off the pale green–and–beige–striped Ralph Lauren sheet and stand. "For now, up you get, ass man. This bedding is going in the wash—and so are you."

CHAPTER 6

THREESOMES

Robbie and I disembark at the Halifax airport. We glance at each other as we ride down the escalator. My parents and older brother will be at the bottom by the baggage carousel. They will have arrived half an hour before us from Calgary, and be standing, smiling, bags in hand. My dad derives great pleasure out of planning trips like this, where we're all coming from different directions and if all goes according to schedule, we fall into formation seamlessly, like a marching band. He has taken 2,542 flights in his life so far and logged them in a journal, including notes on aberrations due to technical difficulties and inclement weather.

One might call it a hobby. Or something else.

This airport makes me feel old. It is miniscule compared to LAX, but once it felt immense. It was here that four-year-old me waited impatiently with my aunt and brother for our parents to return to us from a Bermuda vacation. Here where we greeted my granddad, year after year, waiting to pick us up for Christmas. He is gone now. We moved away from Halifax when I was six—and subsequently moved every few years after that—but returned each year to see my grandparents, aunt, and cousins. In my twenties, Halifax drew me to visit my boyfriend Sam, whose family lives here. We made heartfelt promises that we eventually broke. We made out by the kiosk that sells live lobsters.

As Robbie and I slide off the bottom step, my heart swells when I pick out three smiling faces beaming at us from the small crowd. I let go of Robbie's hand to scurry forward. My mom rushes in, too, while my brother and father hang back. She bounds with her giraffe legs and envelops me in a huge hug. She looks willowy in wide-legged linen pants and a purple t-shirt. It is a wonder that I am related to this group of tall people, all over five-foot-nine, when I stand scarcely five-foot-three. Perhaps my early dalliances with peach schnapps and cigarettes stunted my growth. I breathe in my mom's familiar, sweet perfume.

"We're all here!" she squeals and lets go of me to grab Robbie. I hug my dad and my lanky, red-headed brother, who looks nothing like me. He lifts me a foot off the ground.

"Hiya, Em," he says.

"Hi, Timmy Tim." As he lowers me I notice my dad extend his right hand to Robbie, who moves in for a hug, resulting in a handshake-slash-back-pat move. To say that my British-born father is reserved is a vast understatement. He's met Robbie no fewer than twenty times by now, and I'm certain Rob's petition for my hand in marriage will be met with hearty approval—i.e., two handshakes. Inside, Dad's a pudding, but to the outside world he's, shall we say, rather controlled. The first time he met Robbie's mom and stepdad was at their country house last summer. Dad fell into two feet of water disembarking from a kayak and somehow managed to completely submerge. He popped back out of the lake, brushed a lily pad off his shoulder, righted his sopping-wet hat, and pretended that nothing had happened. Robbie played along and offered him a cold one. I, on the other hand, peed my swimsuit laughing.

"Good to see you guys. I'll go check in with the car rental company, you get your bags, and we'll meet me at the Budget lot?"

"Sure," I say.

"Great, meet you outside," my dad confirms. He and my mom walk off and we three wait for our bags to arrive.

"Ah, Humphrey . . ." Robbie says, referring to my dad. "Maybe one day I'll graduate to the hug."

"Maybe one day Dad will stop wearing Birkenstocks with socks," Tim jokes, and puts one arm around both of us. "This is going to be fun, guys. Family vacation! *Wheee!*" I tilt my head, quizzical at my character-istically deadpan brother's exuberance. "What? It *will* be," he says, then adds in a lowered voice, "I had two rum and cokes on the plane."

"Well, that explains it," I tease. "Hey, when was the last time we went on a trip together, anyway?" I ask.

"Been awhile . . . but this is a first for *you*," he says to Robbie. "The Southwood family bonanza."

"Yup, watch out," I say. "Claire and Hum will go crazy and stay up till nine."

Before long, all six of us are cruising down the highway in a Dodge Caravan with Tim, Robbie, and I giggling in the back. My mom cranes her neck around to figure out what we're on about. We don't really know. Tim's Bacardi buzz is contagious, and we all feel like kids getting away with something. My dad pipes up from the driver's seat: "So, a quick din-ner at the hotel pub and then we'll reconvene in the morning?"

"Sounds good, Dad," I say.

"There's no pressure with plans!" my mom says. "We'll go for dinner with Nanny tomorrow, the rehearsal barbecue dinner is the next night, and then the wedding, but we can spend our days however you want. We can do something together, or go off on our own. Whatever! We're totally easy!!" My mom's adamantly laissez-faire attitude is a response to my dad's hyperorganization. We've based this trip around a family friend's wedding. Aaron, the groom, is my age exactly. His older sister, Laura, is a couple of years older than Tim. Our moms raised us up together in the La Leche League and on home-blended baby food.

It's hard not to spill the beans about being on the marriage bandwagon too. For months now, the secret has been swelling like a balloon stuck on a helium tank. Any minute, I'm bound to fly off the handle, especially now, while I'm feeling giddy with kinship. But Robbie wants to make it official by asking my dad, so I literally bite my upper lip to keep quiet. Plus, I want to avoid any conversations about Robbie's job if I can help it, and that's bound to come up when talk turns to settling down. I mean, that will be one of "the" questions my parents' friends will ask of the groom: "So, what does your future son-in-law do for a living . . . ?" The urge to purge passes.

"I was thinking it might be neat to go to Pier 21," my dad says. "That's where Nanny, Granddad, and I arrived by boat from England in 1952."

"The kids can do whatever they like, Humphrey," my mom says.

"I'd like to see Pier 21," Robbie says.

"Me too," I say. *"Suck up,"* I whisper to Rob.

"Great!" my dad chimes.

"I just want you guys to have a relaxing time while you're here," my mom reiterates.

"Thanks, Mom," I say. "I'm sure we will." I watch the blur of green forest, clapboard homes, and small lakes that line the sleepy highway. The landscape here feels quaint compared to LA. Neither place actually feels like home. Robbie says that home is wherever we are together. I like the sound of that.

Several hours, and a belly full of too rich French onion soup later, I'm reclined on our hotel bed with my legs draped over Robbie. The room is nice, in a petunia-themed kind of way. I'm happy to be stretched out after a long day of travel. He fiddles on his laptop. I absently flip TV channels.

"Canadian TV looks so budget after living in the US," I say. "How is *Little Mosque on the Prairie* still on?" Robbie doesn't answer. "So, my parents brushed by questions about your job pretty quickly?"

"Yeah," he says. "I guess nobody wants to hear about the latest threesome."

"Is that what you filmed yesterday?"

Robbie is silent for a protracted thirty seconds, as is often the case when he's half engaged in something else. I'm not sure whether he's heard me, so I rock my legs over his to remind him I'm here. "What? Threesome, yeah," he eventually says. "At Naughty America. It was pretty vanilla."

"Right, because threesomes are like second base to you." As it comes out, I realize it's not clear whether I'm referring to the show. Forget threesomes, it's known between us that Robbie had a foursome once, whereas I've stuck to one person at a time. He fooled around with a prior girlfriend of his, her roommate, and another guy. Once more, he's a step ahead of me with a point of sexual comparison. If we were ever to venture into threesome or foursome territory (and I'm making zero promises), I'd be the newbie. I can get into the idea as a fantasy, but I'd be worried about the logistics. For one, that I'd lose interest too quickly and be stuck watching Robbie and so-and-so get it on. Second, that my propensity for jealousy might make such a scenario excruciating—which I'm pretty sure is typical threesome fear number 1. Robbie likes to joke that I could only ever have a threesome with two guys who were entirely focused on me because I'd want all the attention. He's probably not wrong. Which begs the question: Do I believe that I'm the most attractive, enigmatic woman out there, capable of captivating such interest? Hardly. But I still want his attention all for myself. I wonder if I was this much of an attention whore back in the sandbox. I'll have to ask Aaron and Laura.

"Do you think watching so much porn is making you kind of numb to it all?" I ask him, as I absently flip through the entire roster of channels again.

"Definitely to mainstream," he sighs. "It's so repetitive."

"Do you watch much porn on your own lately?" I ask, as if it's a nothing question, but the thought instantly makes me feel anxious. I'm too fucking nosy for my own good. And I don't know why I'm going there. We're on our first vacation with my family—clearly the perfect time to discuss porn a little more, now that we're finally away from it. He looks over at me instead of the computer. I stay fixed on the TV screen, chewing my lip.

"Hardly ever," he says. "I get my fill at work." He pauses. "Yes, I used to watch it more occasionally, but we've talked about this. What does it matter, anyway? It's not a big deal."

"Dunno, just curious," I say. But now, since I've already opened Pandora's box of goodies, I have trouble not rifling through the whole thing for loose change. Yes, I know he watches porn, and yes, we've talked about this in the recent past, but Robbie has used this "occasionally" descriptor before, and I've always felt it was a way of glossing things over. It's a wiggle word, and I tend to like clarity when it comes to my understanding of others—especially when it comes to the man I'll be waking up to the rest of my life.

"So how much does 'occasionally' really mean?" I probe.

"I don't know. Sometimes every day, but not always."

"Right, you're the one who thinks every day is occasional," I say sarcastically. Robbie takes me literally.

"It wasn't every day, all of the time, Emily. I could go weeks at a time watching none. What I meant, whenever I said that, was that it wasn't something consistent. It still isn't."

"Oh." I stare at the TV, unable to look at him.

"Why does it make a difference how often I watched it or continue to watch it?" he snaps. He's silent for a minute and then closes his laptop. "It doesn't affect my relationship with you or how much I desire you, which is a lot," he says more gently.

"You don't think porn affects the way you see sex or me at all?"

Robbie sighs. "Do we really have to do this again, right now?"

"I was just curious," I lie. I swing my legs off of him and stand up. "I'm going to take a quick bath."

Sequestered in four bathroom walls, I turn on the water, strip down, and recline into the tub. My ass sticks on the slip-proof, flower-patterned adhesive stickers. I sit awkwardly hunched, tummy divided into two six-inch Subway sandwich rolls, waiting for the water to cover me. What am I trying to get at by bringing this up again? Would I be happier if Robbie didn't like or watch porn as Sam used to claim—true or false? And if I really don't like the truth, then what exactly do I plan to do about it? Find the other non-porn-watching guy in North America and marry him instead? Or ask Robbie to stop watching it for me? I don't want to be the kind of girl who puts out such ultimatums or, for that matter, needs them to feel secure. Would I be happier if I lived in a porn-free world? I've never considered myself conservative, but whenever I think about porn on a personal level—Robbie watching it, filming it, making comparisons based on it—my feelings betray my politics. The water is up to my waist. I turn it off and submerge my head. With my eyes shut, I let my hair swirl over my face, momentarily eclipsing me.

As it turns out, if I based my marriage requirements on a man's porn-watching habits, I'd never reach the altar. When the University of Montreal attempted to conduct a study of twenty-something men who did not watch porn, they couldn't find any. Not a one among them. Arguably, most guys watch porn these days, as do an increasing number of women (one in three, says a recent *Oprah* study). Most adolescents today have exposure to porn by age eleven (so says *New York Magazine*). We are a XXX-consuming culture. And these days, our consumption happens largely via the Internet.

I didn't have much exposure to pornography until into my twenties. Why's that again? Well, for one thing, I was always under the impression that my deceased relatives could see me masturbate. I didn't believe in God's judgment per se, but somehow Great-Aunt Molly's scornful, post-mortem gaze was enough to keep me chaste. Or at least keep me covert. For years I only ever pleasured myself while pretending to be doing something else—like intently studying the Periodic Table, listening to Nirvana on my yellow Walkman, or composing a love poem in hot pink ink. It was no small theatrical task. Overtly sexual material was obviously out of the question.

Elsewhere, VHS had made XXX widely available to inquiring minds in the '80s and '90s, and the Internet was burgeoning with smut. But my girlfriends never shared or talked about salacious material.

Maybe they, too, were superstitious and secretly puritanical. Either way, I was more preoccupied with doodling boys' names in hearts. Finding my way behind the beaded curtain at the local video store or using a dial-up connection for a forty-minute download wasn't on my radar back then. Robbie, on the other hand, with the help of his older brother, ran a small business of recording back-to-back skin flicks onto ninety-minute VHS tapes and selling them to his cohorts at boys' school. Where there's a will there's always a way. Porn and aspiring entrepreneurs have always been close friends.

As an adult with Internet porn readily available, I still deferred to the sexual imaginings in my head. I imagined real people. Say, the weirdly attractive, gold-capped-toothed Italian cashier at the corner store taking me in the cold room against twelve-packs of beer. *Crash. Bang. Boom.*

So it was that up until this point in my life, twenty-eight, I had been more affected by porn via the people I was intimate with than via my own personal consumption. This amplified my feelings that porn was something only for guys. It is hard to say whether I would have taken a personal interest in it long before had I been a postmillennial teen, and how that would have affected me. As it happened, I was late to the buffet table, whether by virtue of timing, gender, or personality. And I felt left out. (There were other reasons I felt like an outsider to porn—i.e., that most of it was still produced by men with a male audience in mind.) But initially, I simply felt left out of a part of Robbie's life. I wanted *all* of the man I was in love with. I was sexually possessive to the nth degree, emotions spawned from my hearty fixation with romantic love, yet willfully repressed by my ironic sensibility and my awareness that it wasn't terribly flattering to behave like Glenn Close in *Fatal Attraction*. Thus we were enmeshed in a jealousy-inducing threesome—him, porn, and me. Porn, the other lover. Porn, the office temptress in red stilettos hovering by the water cooler. Why would he want to get with that nasty-ass ho when he could be with yours truly?

Clearly, I was the victim of a fabricated betrayal. Despite being more open than past boyfriends, he had understandable reservations about sharing certain information with me. Nobody likes to feel judged or monitored, especially in the sexual arena, extra especially by a woman who looks suspiciously like she stars in *True Blood*. I sensed that Robbie had walls up. He sensed that I wanted something more from him—just basically, you know, *everything*. A fool could see I wasn't as comfortable as I feigned to be. We sidestepped in tune to a typical dance of the sexes—woman probes, man shuts down. I stifled a weighty question.

"Um, babe, can I be everything to you sexually forever and ever?"

He repressed a blunt response.

"No, sugarplumbean, you cannot."

It didn't occur to me then that I might not want to be everything to anyone sexually. Or, conversely, that I didn't really want to depend on someone to meet my every need. For the moment, I was still dancing with my private delusions to an old teenage pop song with a dreamy notion—that sex necessarily equates to love.

There is no question that greater access to XXX is changing our sexual development as teens and adults. But how exactly? I like to think our new reality could actually create more equanimity between the sexes. Much depends on how we continue to consume, think, and talk about porn. These are now what I consider productive feminist conversations to be having, rather than my former knee-jerk reactions to porn as inherently good or bad. Neither Robbie nor I was right or wrong. We came from different upbringings, experiences, and comfort levels. We were both entitled to our feelings. Unfortunately for us, entitlement in sex, love, and marriage isn't a sentiment that gets you very far.

Two nights later we're at the rehearsal BBQ dinner in Aaron and Laura's backyard where we used to play all day in the tree house. The scene is casual—a mix of generations in summer pastels. Men hover by the barbecue. Women coo over the token baby. A dog scrounges for scraps on the ground.

After a few speeches are given and burgers and potato salad consumed, the night seems to be winding down. I sip a glass of wine at the perimeters of a conversation with new acquaintances. It's 8:00 PM, and the bride and groom have now departed, sagely resting up for tomorrow. Despite how little we've done today—a bit of shopping and lunch by the harbor—I, too, feel ready for bed. I wander over to my mom and dad, who are chatting with Aaron's mom.

"Ready to go, Emmeau?" My dad asks. He gives me a soccer coach–like pat on the back.

"Yup," I say.

"Why don't you round up the guys and we'll drive back to the hotel." I leave them to their conversation. I can't spot Tim and Robbie anywhere outside, so I head through the backdoor of the house. True to form, I find them in the kitchen drinking gin with some British cousins of the groom. The cousins are clearly a few to the wind, and Robbie and Tim are catching up.

"Mom and Dad are ready to go," I whisper to Tim.

"Already?" he says.

"Yeah, I guess it's winding down."

"Not here. These guys are hilarious," he says. On cue, the small crowd erupts in joyous laughter. I decide it's better not to argue, and wait for Mom and Dad to come through the house instead. Ten minutes and several Cockney-accented inside jokes later, they do.

Back at the hotel, we all board the elevator and say our goodnights.

Mom and Dad debark on the second floor and Robbie, Tim, and I continue to the third. Tim turns to Robbie as we walk down the corridor and says, "I'm going to grab money and a jacket. Meet you guys back downstairs in five?"

"What?" I say.

"Tim wants to go out," Robbie says. "Let's go! It will be fun."

"I don't know," I say. "I'm kind of exhausted."

"I'll convince her," he says to Tim. We continue on down the hallway to our room. I really don't want to go out right now. But I don't particularly want to be alone either. Tomorrow is the wedding and also, coincidentally, my twenty-ninth birthday. Tomorrow is party time; tonight I just want to cuddle and relax.

"You know you want to," Robbie says. "Don't be a downer."

"Don't you want to stay here with me?" I say, leaning in for a suggestive kiss-slash-grope. We make out for a second but Robbie pulls away.

"I promised Tim. Just come, we don't have to stay out forever."

I raise my eyebrows at him. With the state both of them are in, I don't see anyone coming home before last call. "I don't want to go," I say.

"Okay, can I still go?"

Christ, this question. There is no way I'm going to say no. It's like asking me if he can film porn: I want to say no, so obviously I say: "Yeah, have fun. Don't wake me up when you get in." And like that, he's gone.

I strip down and climb into my pajamas. Then I put on the in-room coffeemaker to heat water for tea. This is fine. We can do separate things, no biggie. I flip through TV channels and nosh the remainder of a chocolate bar I bought at LAX. But I'm distracted by old nostalgic thoughts, namely one: Sam. Sam's parents live in Halifax and he comes here every summer for vacation. Being here inevitably makes me think of him.

Robbie has never met Sam. When Robbie and I started seeing each other, Sam and I had recently reconnected and were deciding whether or not to give it another go. More accurately, I was trying to win him back after years of being broken up and realizing how few people there are out there that you really connect with. On his part, Sam was occasionally sleeping with me, but it might have been more like hate-fucking. He still had a chip on his shoulder from when I'd shattered his heart into small shards. So, for a few months before Robbie and I made any commitments, I saw both of them. I was up-front with Robbie about what was going on. Still, it was logistically and emotionally messy and didn't continue for long. Miraculously, we never all ran into each other, even though Montreal is a smallish city. Tonight Robbie is going to meet Sam, through the mutual link of my brother—I am suddenly, utterly, psychically convinced.

This inkling hits me like a shot of adrenaline. I want the whiskey Tim and Robbie are likely consuming. Instead, I have the weather channel and chamomile tea. It is just like me to decide to stay home and then, upon being left alone, feel left out and want to go out. I am the poster girl for reverse psychology. Not to mention a crazy-ass megalomaniac of the astrological sign Leo. But more importantly, is my Sam intuition on point?

I can picture the two of them sitting at a dimly lit bar. They are making small talk, sipping frosty pints of beer, and, of course, comparing notes on me.

"So, you're marrying Emily?" Sam says.

"Yeah, I gather you guys dated for four years?" Robbie returns.

"Yup, best of luck to you." Raises his glass. They clink mugs.

"Thanks, man. She was going to come out tonight but she wasn't up for it." He sips his beer. "You know how she can be."

"What—changeable? Emotional? Not Em," Sam says.

"Yeah, that's an understatement."

"Let me guess: your relationship started out fun and detached and then, *wham*, you were up to your eyeballs in her issues?"

"Something like that," Robbie says.

"What can you do? Bitches are all crazy when the lights come on." Mutual chuckle. "Whiskey?"

"Sure, bro. Why not." Robbie says.

"It's on me—a wedding gift. Hey, by the way, does she still sleep in that hideous old nightgown of her grandmother's?"

Robbie nods.

"Dude, burn it."

Okay, so they're probably not going there. But still, I've enjoyed the tidy compartmentalization of exes that moving across the continent has given us. I appreciate the ability to purge emotional baggage along with one's mismatched socks. I think I only really, truly got over Sam when I left Montreal and all its relationship reminders. And I am over him. But my inner control freak doesn't love the idea of the two loves of my life yucking it up. While all is resolved now, the muddled past was only a few years ago. Must it conjoin on barstools?

I pace the ten steps from the putrid floral loveseat by the window to the DO NOT DISTURB sign on the door. If only I could stop torturing myself. In my frenzy, I bang my shin on the bedframe and sit down in pain. The last time I saw Sam was the summer just before Robbie and I moved away for grad school. I was here in Halifax visiting family and Sam was here too. We were just friends by then; we went swimming in a nearby lake and met up at night for a beer on the patio of a local brew-pub. It was fine, amicable, akin to two old pals with no romantic baggage shooting the shit. About midnight, he excused himself to make a booty call. I was old news—just the ex with nothing more to offer. I took a cab back to Nanny's old-age home where I was staying in the visitors' guest room. Inside, I sat on the slippery polyester bedspread and cried. The door we'd left cracked open for so long was finally shut. Perhaps my fiancé hobnobbing with my old boyfriend is just another nostalgic reminder that my current life decisions are permanent. You know, like death. It's not that I want to be with Sam exactly. It's that I'll never be with anyone else but Robbie. Am I ready for this?

Unlike the throbbing pain in my leg that was there thirty seconds ago and is now forgotten, old emotions can be called up instantly and feel immediate again. I repeatedly dream that Robbie has left me or cheated on me, and worse, fallen out of love. I plead with him, scream, pound on his chest, demand answers, but he simply doesn't care. My ferocity is not just about being betrayed, but about having no emotional hold over him. No power. Zero control. I wake furious and he is unaware, drooling on the pillow. I'm quite sure any old analyst would reckon I have some unaddressed control issues. Or maybe these dreams are manifestations of my own anxieties about everlasting commitment. These days, I feel at once secure and extremely vulnerable. I've never had this much to lose. And I'm worried I'll somehow fuck it right up.

This wee panic attack must be just that, a collection of unconscious, nebulous fears. I feel left out of something completely imagined, just as I have so many times in LA. How is it that I'm here, in my hometown, with my family, managing to feel the same? I pull back the comforter on the bed and lie down, bringing my knees into my chest in a yogic self-hug. The digital clock reads 12:15 AM. Happy goddamned birthday, me. *You're twenty-nine now, Emily. For Christ's sake, learn to self-soothe. It doesn't matter if they meet each other. In fact, you know they'll get along swimmingly; they're both great people, and you're engaged to the man who's right for you. Now stop your lunatic imaginings and go to bed.*

At four in the morning, Robbie comes in, stumbles, and lands in a heap on the bed.

"Hi," I say, instantly pulled from my restless half-sleep.

"Hey," he says. "You're awake."

"Yeah, how was your night?"

"Fun, you'll never believe who I met."

"Sam?"

"Yeah, how did you know? Did you talk to him?"

"No, just a guess."

"You're a witch."

"Possibly," I say. "Was it fun?"

"Yeah, he seems cool. We did shots of whiskey together and then went for Donairs, then we lost him on the street somehow. The police showed up for some bar fight and everyone dispersed . . ." he trails off as he rises and stumbles to the bathroom. I hear him pee, brush his teeth, and get water. Then he flops back into bed. "I can't believe I finally met him. Weird that you didn't come out," he says.

"Yup, weird," I say. "I guess I wasn't supposed to be there. Did you tell him about your job?" Robbie responds with a grunt that is more Neanderthal than English. I look over and he is passed out in all his clothes. Just me and him. Him and me. This is our future.

The next night, our trip culminates at Aaron's sunset wedding reception overlooking Halifax harbor. Up until now, it's been a brutal birthday, between Robbie's and Tim's wretched hangovers and my behaving like an insolent child. But we all pulled it together midday and put on our formal wear. Now, after tearfully witnessing my childhood friend walk the aisle and subsequently shotgunning three flutes of champagne over dinner,

I'm back to my old jovial self. We didn't want to steal any of Aaron's thunder pre-wedding, but with everyone now dancing to Michael Jackson and heavily imbibing, Robbie's ready to make his move.

I'm chatting with my mom on the side of the dance floor when I spot Robbie sidle up to my dad with a scotch in each hand. My dad smiles, nods, and takes a glass. Together, they exit the reception hall onto the waterfront veranda. My stomach flutters and I feel tears welling up again. Wow, I didn't expect to be so moved by this traditional gesture. My knees threaten to buckle, and not just because I've once again made the mistake of wearing four-inch heels to a mostly standing event. I bite the inside of my cheek hard and continue nodding along faux-intently to my mom's chatter about whether or not to go on a yoga retreat with some retired friends.

Two minutes later, they walk back in. Dad beams. Robbie fires me a redundant thumbs-up sign as they walk toward us.

"Well, we'll have another wedding to attend in the near future, Claire," Dad says to Mom.

"What? *Really!!?*" she squeals. "I knew it!" she envelops me, and then Robbie, in an asphyxiating hug. Then she cozies up to Dad and locks arms with him. They look elated, proud.

"Did he hug you?" I whisper to Rob, as we move to stand side by side. He takes my hand in his and squeezes it.

"Nope," he whispers back. "But he did a fist pump. Twice."

Two weeks later in Montreal, Kate and I are numerous cocktails into a catch-up marathon on her backyard terrace. The humid night air is thick with the smell of cut grass and our cigarette smoke. Montreal always makes me want to light up. I blame French Canadians for continuing to make cancer look cool.

"Okay, I have to say something," Kate blurts sometime around midnight. We have both sufficiently imbibed enough to feel pleasantly buzzed, and we've covered all the obvious topics—my engagement, her recent horse show and man drama. "I might be totally off base here," she says, "but I've thought about it, and if things were the other way around, I'd want you to be straight with me."

"What is it?" I say.

"Especially now that you're getting married."

"Jesus, you're kind of scaring me." I put down my glass on the patio table and light another cigarette to brace myself for whatever she's going to share.

"I was having drinks with Rebecca last week and she mentioned that Robbie had hooked up with a girlfriend of hers in New York." She pauses, takes in my petrified expression, and immediately begins to backpedal. "But you know, she said it was a few years back, and I'm sure it was before you guys were serious. Oh crap, I should shut up."

"Who was the girl?" I say with the determination of a customs officer.

"I've never met her, just some friend of Rebecca's from her time at McGill."

"That sounds like dumb gossip." I swirl the ice cubes in my drink, creating a tornado of watery vodka and squashed limes.

"You're probably right. I'm sorry I brought it up. It just seemed like maybe the kind of thing you should know. I didn't want you to hear it from someone else or find out, you know, later on."

"I'm sure it's nothing," I say. I feel defensive. I don't like the suggestion that people know things about my fiancé that I don't. Is he hiding something from me? How recent was this alleged hookup? We've talked about the on-again-off-again period in our relationship, and Robbie has always said he wasn't with anyone else, even though we weren't entirely committed. What about while we lived long distance? My stomach is suddenly sloshing with alcohol and doubt. I fiddle with the engagement ring—two diamonds flanking a ruby—that is now adorning my left hand. The ring even came with a declaration: during a visit to his parents the other day, Robbie perched on one knee in his mother's kitchen and told me he wants to live his whole life with me. Yup, jealous, unstable me. Things felt concrete, real, optimistic, until a few seconds ago.

"Fuck, should I not have said that? I shouldn't. I'm sorry," she says, taking in my grey pallor. She puts her hand on my knee. "Are you okay?"

"It's not exactly what I want to think about right now, but I'll talk to him about it." Unfortunately he's not here to talk to. He's back in LA filming porn.

After trying to negotiate spending time with his family as well as catching up with my girlfriends, we decided that I would stay on in Montreal and even scout a few wedding locations for next summer. He had to get back to work filming *On Fire*—a porno starring twenty men madly fucking on a fire truck. You know, the usual. I wish that I could rewind a week to celebrating our engagement, clinking glasses of champagne with my soon-to-be in-laws. But we're not in Kansas anymore. He's off filming *The Wizard of Ass*.

Kate and I finish our drinks. I refuse to let my mind completely unravel before I know the facts. My cell phone is nearly drained, so I tell her I'm going to make my call in her office and not to wait up. I have zero plan of attack. I dial.

"Have you been with anyone else since we've been together?" I launch with.

"Hey, it's late in Montreal. What's going on?"

"Just answer the fucking question."

"Why are you asking me this?"

"Because."

"I don't understand why you're calling me up with accusatory questions." He is clearly pissed by the sidelong attack, but I persist.

"Have you? Since you've been with me?"

"Please don't do this. We don't go digging around in each other's past, Emily. That's not our style."

"Answer me!"

Robbie is silent, and I realize I'm scribbling furiously on the Post-it in front of me. It looks like a lie detector gone haywire. "Are you sure you want to know?" he says.

"So, *yes?* The answer is yes?"

He pauses. "Yes. It was before we were serious. That week I went to New York. Things weren't that great between us, so I didn't tell you."

"No, instead you told me that you'd only been with *me* since the first time we slept together! You've always been so fucking insistent about that! Why did you lie? I was honest with you about still seeing Sam!" I am crying now and can barely make out my words.

"We just fooled around. We were really drunk. Can we talk about this in person?"

"Who is she?"

"Just an acquaintance."

"Well, other people know! She told Rebecca, who told Kate. I had to hear about it from my maid of honor!"

"I'm so sorry you found out this way. It didn't mean anything. I was really struggling with you not letting me in back then." We are both silent for a minute.

"I need to tell you something else," Robbie says. "That week when you broke up with me I had a one-night stand with the girl I was dating before you. It was stupid, I . . ."

I hang up and slide from the chair onto the carpet. He calls right back. I lift the receiver and place it down again, then leave it off its cradle. I can't hear any more, not a word. So this is what actual betrayal feels like. Curled in the crook of Kate's pressboard IKEA desk with the muffled sound of the dial tone above me, I close my eyes and sob.

CHAPTER 7

COUPLES

Among all the crude categories on YouPorn, "couples" is downright quaint. Two people, presumably in some kind of relationship, have sex. It's almost hard to imagine that being anyone's fantasy anymore. Except for the fact that it prevails as the most common cultural desire. We mostly aspire to couple up. We typically go two-by-two to the bedroom, to the altar, and we're skeptical of those who don't—swingers, spinsters, Mormons. We don't, by and large, live in polyamorous relationships, despite the frequent media chatter about new types of unions. Is this slowly changing? We often hear the platitude that monogamy between two people is not natural. There's plenty of proof to suggest it's broken—like the Ashley Madison tagline "Life is short. Have an affair." But if monogamy between two people is flawed, then what is the ideal arrangement?

When Robbie told Michel I was having trouble with the content of the show he said, "Why? It's just sex." Well, touché, Michel. I have heaped plenty of emotional baggage on sex in the past. Too much, perhaps. I'm going to go ahead and blame oxytocin, the love hormone we release when we orgasm. That combined with too many viewings of *The Notebook* and perhaps a dash of the biological urge to tame me a good man. I don't rationally think that sex and love always have to be connected.

Experience has shown me they are not, for I've tussled in the sheets with people I did not love and folks who didn't love me. It's also my understanding that sometimes the desire to have more than one partner is just about sex. Nothing more. Moreover, I don't believe a relationship need always screech to a halt with a sexual dalliance as it does on *Days of Our Lives*. Incidentally, I've also discovered people don't regularly come back from the dead either. Who knew?

The trouble is that sex and emotions aren't always easy to unbraid, especially, though it hurts my egalitarian brain to say so, for women. Whether this is because of nature or nurture, I can't say. But it seems to be the way it is. *Or at least the way I am, dearest Michel.* At times I think it would be handy if I could just axe jealousy and possessiveness from sexual relationships. Maybe such an emotional compartmentalization can be learned. In fact, I occasionally believe that I could learn to operate that way. Still, if I learned to be 100 percent nonpossessive, I question whether I'd be left with a relationship compromised in other ways. Jealousy may be necessary for me to, *you know*, care. How do you discover your perfect ratio? How do you measure it faultlessly, like baking powder, to not have the whole thing collapse in on itself? What if something like this happens?

ME: "Darling, can you pick our son up from daycare tomorrow?"

HUSBAND: "Tomorrow? Shit, I was planning to act out a scene from *Fifty Shades of Grey* with my new lover. And I have to pick up Jimmy Choo's, some silk ties, and a couple butt plugs after work. Can you fetch him?"

ME: "Seriously? You're buying her *Jimmy Choo's?* I want a divorce."

Okay, that's a dumb example. You'd obviously have a "no gifts" clause in an open relationship, among other things, like no kissing or anal or whatever is designated just for you and your sweetie. You have to be businesslike, sensible, not whimsical and romantic. Blowjobs, not luxury women's wear, Emily—*duh.*

I recently read the Arianne Cohen article "Asking for It," about her nonmonogamous relationship. It sounded like a mature, organized, and rational arrangement that she came to when she discovered the joys of having multiple no-strings-attached "playmates," as well as waking up with a primary mate to do the crossword with. As I read her descriptions, I remembered the lure of new sex. I could definitely see the appeal. Until she offered up this line, three-quarters of the way through the article: "It was messy sometimes—new, open relationships always are, because you only learn what your boundaries are from your partner's stabbingly painful trial and error—but things stabilized."

"Things stabilized." Okay, but that "stabbingly painful" interim period sounds pretty shitty, no? My concern is that such an interim period would last, say, forever. I imagine having my husband over at one of his girlfriends' houses for a romp while I sit at home pounding chips and watching *The Bachelor* and immediately want to off myself. It seems like so much depends on timing, like having him meet a lover just as I meet a lover, and the two of us being interested in our other lovers to more or less the same degree. Is that possible? Plausible? Is it safer to maneuver like the French—don't ask, don't tell—or better to get all hippy-dippy and share *everything*? Ick. The trial and error of it all seems like an awfully big risk. Alas, maybe twenty years of marriage makes this seem worth it. Only time and libidos will tell.

The next morning, I wake up in Kate's bed. As usual, she has already left at 6:00 AM for the stables. I vaguely remember making my way here before dawn and sliding in next to her, as we have on sleepovers since we were fourteen. I go to the bathroom and turn on the shower. In the mirror, my face shows the wreckage. My eyes are swollen. My nose is puffy like I ran headlong into a brick wall. (And I know how that looks because I actually did that once while playing an ill-conceived game of pin the tail on the donkey. Don't ask.) Mascara stains my cheeks. My head threatens to hemorrhage. I pop two Advil, then take a third for good measure, and stand under the stream of hot water. Where does one go from here? This afternoon I'm supposed to be driving back up to Robbie's country house to visit a wedding venue with his mom, his stepfather, and my parents— who are coincidentally here in Montreal visiting old friends. There's no way I can face them all like this. But somehow the prospect of staying here and explaining last night's conversation to Kate sounds just as hard. Since she won't be back from the barn for several hours, I wrap myself in her bathrobe, retrieve my charged cell phone, and climb back into bed. I know I can't avoid Robbie forever. And even though I'm furious, I still feel bad that he is in LA worrying. I decide to call Hilary, who is notoriously nonjudgmental. I need a dose of that right now.

"Hey, Hil, can you talk?" I say when she answers.

"Sure. Are you back in LA? Are you okay?"

"No to both. I had a rough night." I proceed to give her the overview of the situation.

"Wow, okay. First of all, why the hell did Kate tell you that?"

"I don't know. In her own way, I think she meant well. She's protective of me."

"Well, you know now, so there's no going back. From the sounds of it, he slept with the second girl when you broke up with him, which isn't fun to think about. But it's also a pretty natural response to having your heart broken. Weren't you with Sam that week?"

She's right about the week in question. It was during the period when, after several months of dating, Robbie put me on the spot and told me his feelings for me were too strong to do the casual thing anymore. Unprepared to commit at that moment, I told him we should probably stop seeing each other altogether. After just a few days without him in my life, I missed him terribly. I wanted to be with Robbie. I knew then my relationship with Sam was really over. The Robbie "breakup" didn't last long. But clearly much transpired in the interim.

"Yeah, that's true," I say. "I just don't know why he was so adamant about only having been with me since day one. Why lie?"

"Hard to say. He probably just wanted to believe it was pure or something. It can't have been easy for him dealing with you still having feelings for Sam. He probably did it in the first place to bolster his ego, and then felt worse."

"Then there's the New York girl . . ."

"Which is shitty, but also happened before you guys were really serious. It was probably just a drunken hookup, a fleeting attraction. That whole time was so messy. I remember. It doesn't really count as the beginning of your relationship." She sighs, then continues. "Sometimes I really think we're better off not knowing certain things. There's a grace period at the beginning of any relationship. Robbie adores you, Em. We all know it." Her words make me tear up again.

"I know," I whimper. "I adore him too. I'm a fucking mess, Hil."

"I know, we all are," she says. "We're all works in progress. I don't think this really changes anything."

Is she right? Is everything slightly off-color but basically still the same? We hang up and I take note of the twenty-some missed calls from

Robbie. I still feel miserable, but as anticipated, she provided some perspective. I take a deep breath and dial.

"Hi," he says. He sounds as if he was sleeping but immediately transitions to sounding worried and awake: "Are you going to leave me? Please don't."

"I don't think so," I say.

"I'm so sorry, Emily. I'm sorry I lied to you, and I'm sorry this all came out like this."

"I know," I say, in full-blown tears again. "I didn't need this right now."

"I wish I could be with you. It was all a long time ago now and we weren't where we are now."

"I just wish I didn't have these thoughts in my head." I shudder as I picture Robbie with someone else—someone who looks vaguely like Eva Mendes—fumbling in the dark. Scratch that, screwing with pornographic floodlights on.

"That one-night stand was terrible. I was so upset with you and hurt. I went home with her and then ran out of there in the morning. I just wanted to pretend it never happened and I justified never telling you because we were broken-up."

"I get it, you didn't have to tell me, but you've always been so resolute about never being with anyone else during that time."

"I guess somewhere I kind of wanted to hold the Sam stuff over you. Be better than you were."

"I'm really angry at you right now."

"I know."

"And you're filming porn and I have to go hang out with our parents! How did this happen like this?"

"Don't give up on us," he says. "It might be nice to be in the country with our parents. And at least it's gay porn today," he jokes.

"I think that was supposed to make me feel better."

"No luck?"

"Not yet. I'm going to try and nap."

"Okay, can you call me when you wake up? I mean, only if you want. I love you so much."

"I love you too."

I hang up and burrow myself in a mound of pillows. I'm exhausted. For once, my mind spins for only a few moments before I feel myself drift off.

A few hours later I am on a country road, driving my future mother-in-law's Subaru, which she loaned me for the visit. I listen to the *Forest Gump* soundtrack I find in the glove box and sing aloud to Bob Seger's "Against the Wind." When it ends, I hit Replay. I pound the steering wheel like Tom Cruise in *Jerry Maguire*. I'm definitely running up against some blustery weather. Surely old Bob knows how I feel. Kate came home just before I left, and I told her things are a mess but are going to be okay. She apologized again. It's unsettling to think that she's been questioning Robbie, what, for weeks? Months? My heart hurts. My brain is like an LCD picture frame of tortured images. I really didn't need a literal reason to feel jealous when I'm already so volatile.

I drive. Fast. There is nothing else to do right now but wait. *Feel*—and wait *not* to feel so much. Why did I demand answers from him? Even as a child, I hated being pandered to. I wanted people to speak plainly with me. If there was truth to be heard, I wanted to know it, confront it, no matter how much it hurt. But maybe Hilary is right about sweeping the occasional fact under the rug. My insistence on knowing all the fleshy details so often burns me. Right now, I yearn to know less.

I pull onto the dirt road that leads to the lake house and drive the remaining ten minutes canopied under bright green foliage. As I round a bend, I see the blue lake peeking out through the trees. Soft, humid air comes through the open car window. I bump along half out of my body with fatigue and park in front of the muted blue-green bungalow. I turn the ignition off, climb out of the car onto solid ground, and haul my suitcase out of the trunk.

"Hello-oo!" Robbie's mom singsongs from the kitchen as I walk through the screen door. It clacks shut behind me. "Do you want something cool to drink before we go?" she says as she enters the foyer, looking jovial in capri pants and a coral button-down. I stand dumbfounded. "Are you okay, dear?" she says when she sees my face.

"Yes." I'm already tearing up, so now I have to say something. I can't think of what to make up. "Someone just told me something about Robbie, with someone else, before we were serious," I haphazardly piece together. "It was hard to hear." I let go of my weighty suitcase and it tips over, landing next to my feet.

"Oh, you kids can be so cruel with information," she says with clear disapproval. I ignore the slightly condescending "you kids" because right now I feel like a floundering child who knows nothing about the ways of the world. "Come here." She envelops me in a hug, which is a relief because it means I don't have to look at her while I bite down hard on my lip to contain myself. "Why on earth would someone tell you that?" I can feel her shaking her head. I don't answer. "Well, why don't you put your stuff in your bedroom, freshen up, and we'll go in a few minutes, okay?"

I nod and descend the stairs to the cooler air on the main level. "Your room," she called it. Robbie's room is now my room too. I am a part of the family, dirty secrets and all. The thought makes me tear up again. I sit on the bed for a minute and focus on not crying. Then I take my makeup bag out and attempt to brighten up my face with blush and mascara. The result is a B–. I change from my jean shorts and tank top into a navy and white-flowered summer dress and a pair of wedge sandals. Now I can almost pass for a newly engaged woman. Maybe one who just came off a ten-hour intercontinental flight.

The drive to the inn takes forty minutes, back along the country roads I just maneuvered. I sit in the backseat with my sunglasses on, and Lynn and Roger make chatter, pointing out landmarks here and there. I am thankful to be chauffeured. I'm not quite sure how I managed to drive up here; my adventures on LA freeways must have marginally improved my road skills. My parents, who met in the '70s in Montreal, used to come up here to car rally on these roads. Yup, my rational, business-minded father would spin out of turns and even flip the occasional car. It's hard to believe now. Mom and Dad currently are coming from a nearby friend's country house to meet us. It's just my folks, future in-laws, and me—a bride-to-be, minus her groom. I can't believe we're doing this now, after the night I've just had, but calling the whole thing off would require too much explanation.

We pull up to the blue and white-shuttered inn. My parents are standing in the driveway. I hop out and give them both hugs. It's only been a few days since we parted ways in Halifax but everything feels different. The innkeeper, a man in his sixties who runs the place with his partner, escorts us to the small chapel on the property. I have often imagined our ceremony taking place outside, sky overhead, grass underfoot, but as soon as we enter the chapel, a calm comes over me. The room is lined with wooden pews. Soft light filters through stained-glass windows. While I am not a religious person per se, this place definitely has an "energy." Am I just delirious, hungover, and emotional enough to think I've found God? Not likely. But I like it in here. In fact, I would like to dismiss everyone, curl up on a pew, and take a five-hour nap. My dad comes up next to me and puts his arm around me, pulling me back to reality. "Well, we'd have to remove the cross," he says. Dad is a staunch atheist. I look up and laugh. There is a ten-foot-tall wooden crucifix at the front of the room, as well as several bleeding-Jesus molds here and there. Who am I kidding? He's right; they'd have to go.

"Can we decorate the room as we like?" I ask the owner and he nods. My mom and Lynn burble around the room. Outside, we six walk around to the back of the inn, where a green rolling field unfurls from the hilltop like pie dough. A small lake shines in the meadow below. Great pots of red geraniums and white Adirondack chairs sprinkle the lawn. It's gorgeous. We walk over to the reception hall, which has been built on one side of the inn for hosting weddings, as the innkeeper rambles on about dinner menus, place settings, whatnot. The ambience of the room is typical Quebec countryside–meets–Kellerman's from *Dirty Dancing*. At one end there is a disco ball over a wooden dance floor. Windows looking out to the meadow line the walls. I love it. The four parents whisper to each other, clearly attempting to keep their opinions to themselves, not wanting to influence me. I leave them in the reception hall and walk back out onto the hilltop on my own. I picture all of our friends and family here, a year from now next August. Me in a white dress, maybe off-white, nothing too dramatic or poofy. Robbie in a crisp grey suit. I picture Robbie shagging someone else. I flinch as my mom comes up beside me and grabs my arm.

"So?!!" she says, clearly no longer able to contain herself.

"It's perfect," I say quietly.

"It's only the first place, but it's special, isn't it? Humphrey, she likes it!" she calls out to my dad. Roger and Lynn approach, beaming.

"I thought she might," says Roger, reaching out and squeezing my hand. I catch Lynn giving me a sympathetic smile. She is the only one half aware of the subtext of the day.

We continue our tour around the inn. The interior décor is, shall we say, eclectic. A mishmash of styles and odd paraphernalia—model horses, teacups, one too many fringed lamps. Some might call it junk. But it suits us in a way; the interior contrasts with the exterior. I feel immediately settled on this place. Done. We will marry here, provided our relationship doesn't imminently implode.

"I suppose we'll have to get the groom's opinion? Will he be joining us?" the innkeeper asks, reading my mind.

Nope! He's filming some dudes taking it up the ass on a fire truck! You know—Jet Set, it's a gay porn production house.

Instead I say, "Unfortunately, he's back in LA working."

"Ah, another time."

I nod. Another time indeed.

After the tour, we sit on the hilltop terrace and have a glass of afternoon wine. Thankfully, my sunglasses cover the various waves of emotion that undoubtedly color my face. Sadness. Elation. Skepticism. Faith.

Later that night, I climb under a blue and grey–checkered duvet in one of Robbie's t-shirts. Even though the night air is still warm, I like to sleep under the weight of a cover. My limbs feel leaden. I should call Robbie now and tell him the details of today, but I know speaking with him will awake all of the feelings I want to put to bed. I curl up on the side where he usually sleeps. My mind flitters between thoughts. I watch a firefly light up outside the window, thinking that the weird thing about having your fears manifested is that you don't fall apart. Instead, your body just absorbs the shock.

The next morning I don't want to call Robbie. I have two days to kill before my flight home to LA. It's enough that I'm in his house, surrounded by his things, his world. I take a long swim in the lake with Lynn and a walk through the forest with Roger, listening intently while he points out birds. We drink tea in the afternoon and transition to gin and tonic after that. It feels like a ritual, a WASP family cleansing of sorts. We linger together over dinner, watch some Masterpiece Theatre, and when the day is done, I'm still not ready to talk to Rob. He calls but I ask Lynn to take a message, saying I'll call him after my bath. But I know I won't. I don't really want to hear about porn shoots. I don't care to feel the surges of emotions or further ignite my tortured visualizations. I try to concentrate on just being here, staying upright. I meticulously slice away each noxious thought from my consciousness and toss the moldy ends in the trash. I think that if I focus hard enough on the matters at hand—being the perfect, jovial houseguest!!!—all will be saved. Weirdly, it kind of works. The Victorians were certainly on to something when it comes to keeping up appearances—right now, covering up the raunchy bits seems to help.

The next day, I take a drive to my friend Stephanie's cottage, which is on another lake forty minutes away, and we check out a couple of other wedding venues to at least have a comparison. We lose our way in the countryside searching for a European-themed inn, and drive up and down the same road ten times. When we arrive it looks like *The Sound of Music* threw up all over the hillside. We stifle our giggles as the event's planner shows us around the fake Alps, imagine me walking down the aisle in a dirndl dress, then hit the road. Over ice cream in St. Agathe, I tell Steph the saga of my past week. It sounds better in retrospect than it did a few days ago. Robbie kind of cheated on me! And yup, he's still off filming porn! And I'm hanging out with his parents and planning our quaint country wedding! Ha! *Of course it takes a certain, beleaguered sort of brain to get the full spectrum of humor.* All the same, by the time I drive back to Robbie's country house I feel much more grounded. I fly back to LA tomorrow, but today I am right here. I decide that driving alone in the country should be prescribed for most minor cases of heartbreak. Sometimes a girl just needs to unhinge herself from her significant other, rattle along dirt roads in a hunk of metal, belly stuffed with mocha-fudge ice cream, and remember that she alone is perfectly alright in the world.

The next day, I land back at LAX. Robbie's waiting for me at the airport. I feel like I'm meeting a stranger. I'm nervous. I can tell he is too. We stand hugging each other for a long time before separating.

"Hi," he says. "Do you still like me?"

I nod.

"You like me?" He leans in and kisses me hard. He lifts my bag from my shoulder and we walk toward the parking garage. I spot our pale green Elantra. It's filthy and sports a three-foot scratch on the right side where I recently carved it along our garage wall. It's as scuffed as our relationship at the moment. But it still runs. Robbie opens the passenger door for me, a gesture that always makes me feel special. Lynn raised a polite man. I shudder as I picture him opening the car door for the girl he took home when we were broken-up.

We rattle along the freeway in silence for a few minutes. The radio is turned down, just barely audible, but neither of us moves to turn it up or off. For once, Robbie breaks the silence first as we cruise past downtown.

"What did you think of the inn my folks showed you?" he asks.

"It's amazing," I say, looking at him out of the corner of my eye. He darts me a quick glance and then focuses back on the road, changing three lanes swiftly and merging onto the Hollywood 101.

"Are we going to get married there?" he probes further. He's not really asking about the wedding venue. The subtext is clear to both of us: Can we bridge this unbearable distance between us, which is only the car console but feels like the Pacific? Do you forgive me? And if you do, could you let me know soon so that I can eat and sleep and breathe normally again?

"Yeah, I think we will," I say and place my hand over his on the gearshift. He exhales. I turn the radio up and Fleetwood Mac croons "Sara" while we drive the remaining five miles home.

When we arrive, Matt is in the living room drinking a smoothie and working on his laptop.

"Hey, Emiloo!" he says. "How was your trip?"

"Hi, Matty. Good, thanks. How've you been?"

"You know, hanging out on gay porn sets. Did Robbie tell you about yesterday?" He makes a grimace.

"Don't think so," I say and look to Rob.

"Just a guy who couldn't stay hard, so they wound up injecting something directly into his penis," he says. "And there was another guy doing his first gay porn," Matt continues. He's straight, has a girlfriend, but she doesn't know. *Gay for pay.* Can you imagine?"

Home sweet crass home, I think as I place my laptop bag on my desk by the window. Robbie wheels my suitcase into our room. I know the term Matt's referencing from watching a previous season of *Webdreams,* which followed a married man, who though straight, openly worked in gay porn. His wife would kiss him goodbye as he went off to shag men for money. It was his job, not infidelity by their set of rules. I look at Robbie, now standing in the living room doorway. I wonder whether I could ever be that nonpossessive, open to other lovers *and* genders. Why sure, what's next! Matt types and slurps away.

"Anyone hungry?" I say. "I'm going to walk around the corner and pick up some Thai food."

"Stuffed Chicken Panang for me please," Matt says. I grab my purse.

"Want company?" Robbie asks. I nod. He walks out the door with me and grabs my hand. We walk to the restaurant, discuss what to eat, order, wait in silence. Walk home in silence. We eat in front of the TV out of takeout containers. Then Robbie and I go to our bedroom and undress each other, making out the whole time like when we first fell in love. Our desire is teenage-esque, palpable. I don't think it's just because of the time we've spent apart, although that always helps. Thinking about him with other women has made me jealous. Now I want to know that his desire is for me, that mine is for him. I want bodily evidence, proof. He goes down on me, then I on him, and we wind up in missionary—that old staple, which, despite all the acrobatic fuck Olympics I've been exposed to lately, is still a top pick. I like the weight of him on me. We both cum hard, and then lie still—sweaty, exhausted, tangled up.

In this moment, he is mine, I am his; there is no doubt.

CHAPTER 8

AMATEUR

My job is becoming problematic. Contracts trickle in, and besides being in the midst of the biggest economic meltdown since the Great Depression, I suspect that I'm not very good at corporate writing. Hence the degrees in poetry, not business. Seriously, did I really think palindromes would pay the bills? What kind of crack was I smoking? Some good crack, apparently. Oopsie. Oh well. Moving on. I start looking for something else in my downtime, which is suddenly *all the time.* Robbie and I knew that when I moved here it would be harder for me to bring in the big bucks because of my limited visa situation. Basically, according to the Department of Homeland Security, I'm only allowed to work for this one employer (who, okay, if I'm laying it all out there, happens to be my future brother-in-law). I can look for a new employer who'll sponsor me. But who would hire me—a generally unqualified illegal alien—without some sort of nepotistic drive? Why wouldn't they hire an American with two equally remote degrees? One of the many, many currently out-of-work Americans? Why, they *would*. Which makes my job search as fruitful as panning for gold in the LA River.

My voicemail remains empty. My email collects spam about penile implants. Needless to say, Robbie is pulling in more money than I am these days and paying for more of our living expenses. After years of making my own way in the world, it feels strange to be partially supported. He isn't putting any pressure on me. His take is magnanimous: what's mine is yours. Still, I do a good job of putting pressure on myself. I've never thought of myself as the "kept woman" type. Much as I feign to be Betty fucking Crocker from time to time, I don't think it actually suits me.

I have an interview for a job as a part-time English tutor. It goes well but would entail me driving out to Malibu several times a week, just for a few hours. The gas money and time in traffic don't make it viable. Not to mention I don't have consistent access to a car. Nor is my brother-in-law all that psyched about having me bill "miscellaneous services" through his company. This was another bad idea. I keep looking.

Hilary says she can probably hook me up with a waitressing job if I'm interested. She lives above a restaurant on Sunset Boulevard that might, *ahem*, hire me under the table. Do I want to waitress again? Not really. It feels like a step backward. Yet my student debts loom large. Yes, not only did I acquire useless degrees, I paid through the nose for them. Always thinking, that's me! Every day after fruitless Internet job searches, I consider dropping my resumé at the restaurant. Maybe it would be good to have a social type of job. I imagine making martinis along with small talk. I could smile, laugh, and pour! Satisfy gastronomical whims, clad in an ill-fitting cocktail dress with lychee juice up to my armpits and a secret wish to poison my patrons. Who am I kidding? I hate waitressing as much as the next poet. I tell myself a daily mantra—you moved here in support of Robbie's job and if you were back in Canada things would be different. You'd be a poorly paid administrative assistant, no problemo!

I keep looking for work and planning the wedding. I write the odd bit of clichéd verse, bake pies using a Cindy Crawford recipe I learned on *Oprah,* and endeavor to stay positive.

Robbie and I are sitting on the lawn one day after work drinking Coronas. It is September but hot as July. His recently shaved head rests on my thigh. I run my hand over it, lingering on the baby-soft fuzz where he's balding.

"*Mmm,* more," he says. I scratch harder with my stress-bitten fingernails.

"How did today go?" I ask. We've actually gone several weeks without discussing porn. I've been wrapped up in my work search and remarkably mute after all the Montreal drama. But today I feel calm, collected, and I want to propose something to him.

"Fine," he says. "It's getting so boring."

"Hey, do you think Michel's offer to get me on set still stands?" I ask. "I've been thinking maybe I could write an article about it. It could pay something!" (Side note: Only poets consider freelance journalism a step up in pay.)

"Maybe. I'll ask him."

"Thanks!" I say. "I think being able to see how things work for myself could be really good, don't you? And then maybe I could write some kind of women's perspective about seeing the inner workings of the porn world!"

"Yeah, maybe."

"You don't think so?" I stop scratching his head and wait for his answer.

"No, I guess it could be," he says, and rubs his head against my fingertips. I halfheartedly begin scratching again, feeling a little deflated by his lackluster response. Is he worried about me seeing what he sees? Worried that I can't handle it? Maybe he just doesn't want me around?

"Well I think it would really help and possibly be fruitful, writing-wise. Where were you guys today? Could I have been there?" I ask.

"I'm not sure. We were at Naughty America again, filming a five-girl lesbian scene."

"Hot lesbians?"

"Yeah, pretty hot," he admits.

"Oh yeah, anyone in particular?" I blurt without thinking and quickly realize my question sounds like a loaded gun. Robbie pauses for a minute, sips his beer.

"Eva Angelina is sexy."

"Well, don't forget to ask Michel for me." I lean back on the grass and stare up at the tall palms. Immediately I wonder what Eva looks like. Fucks like. What her life is like. Does she enjoy what she does? I guess I haven't changed all that much.

The next day I type "Eva Angelina" into Google. Her website comes up. She has dark brown hair, looks Latina or maybe part Asian, is voluptuous (naturally?). She wears glasses and copious iridescent plum eye shadow. In her photo gallery, she is smiling while holding cocks up to her mouth or getting penetrated in various ways. She looks happy. She has a tribal tattoo on her lower back. Wikipedia tells me she was born in 1985 (only seven years younger than I!) and that she's Cuban, Chinese, and Irish. Neato.

I sit back in my chair. I like that she's not stick-thin. I like her nerdy glasses. Then the thought of Robbie filming her and feeling attracted to her bubbles up. Why can't I find that a turn-on? Or at least feel neutral. I close my computer. Go take a bath.

I repeat this behavior several times over the next week. Sometimes searching for her, sometimes other people he films: Johnny Gun and his pornstar girlfriend. Paris, the young webcam girl who he says is high maintenance. She has bad skin up close. Madison X, the lesbian fetishist whose husband films and directs her. She wears a lot of cheesy latex. A shit ton of eyeliner. I scrutinize each of them. Despite sitting at my computer daily, this is the first time that I've actually looked any of them up. Until now, they've existed only in my head.

Feeling brave from my confrontations, I go to YouPorn and peruse the thumbnail video captions. There's "chicks who drink dicks"; "big tit teen gets fucked on her bed"; "Japanese hottie takes multiple creampie." So many stellar choices! I click on "Latina cutie wants big cocks," and in a few seconds, boy is she getting her fill. She's hot, minus the heavily sedated expression. Bald cha cha, of course. Some tats. The two guys going to town on her, however, are *not* my idea of eye candy. Their members, as advertised, are freaking enormous, which merely elicits a fear of vulvodynea. They walk right at her from off camera, dick first, and ram her pussy, mouth, then ass. The whole time saying shit like "Yeah baby, suck that. You love that. *Oooh,* take it." I cringe. PLEASE SHUT UP! But despite my critiques, I'm turned-on by watching people, yup, even these folks, have sex. *Huh, who knew my libido could override my running editorial? I guess that's what the masses are on about.* With my right hand down my jean shorts, I cum in about three seconds, no vibrator required—wow, it's been years since I left old Sancho in the bedside drawer! Then I close the window and proceed to stuff my face with three pieces of last night's reheated pizza.

By day three of this routine, I've made a discovery. I like lesbian porn! Yeah, I dig girls sometimes, but mostly I'm sick of these monster ginormo-cocks that appear out of absolutely nowhere. Where do they come from? It's just too damn much surprise cock, people! To boot, these dudes look absolutely nothing like anyone I would care to be with. They are all muscle, in the manner indicative of steroid abuse, and all appear to have been freshly dipped in a vat of canola oil. *Is it too much to ask for an awkward but sexy fellow, say, pulled off the street in Williamsburg? Why hasn't anyone thought about cruising around in a dude-banging bus there? I bet the gays have . . . I should look.* Anyway, there seems to be much, much more foreplay in lesbian porn. The scenarios presented are just as dumb and poorly acted—hottie masseuse goes downtown on busty patient. But at least there's some context. I like context—call me a cliché girl. I also like seeing women being pleasured in ways other than repeat penetrations—kissing, boob fondling, hand jobs, cunnilingus. And at least this genre starts with some gentle fingering before busting out the giant strap-ons. Personally, I don't like walking out of the shower and getting slapped in the face by a ten-inch cock, any more than I like bending down to fetch some carrot sticks from the crisper and getting rammed in the ass. Call me crazy. So yup, lesbo porn! Who knew that was my thing?

Masturbation used to be more of an event for me. I'd retreat to the bedroom and recline with old Sancho, a glass of Shiraz, some Sade, and a fantasy like Bradley Cooper going down on me while Channing Tatum feeds me dark chocolate and sucks on my nipples. Okay, maybe no Sade. But anyway, the whole process used to take at least five minutes. Now, with this whole YouPorn discovery, I'm done in under thirty seconds! Occasionally, the selection of a suitable clip takes me a little longer. Like yesterday, when I stumbled upon a particularly old suburban MILF seducing a pubescent tween on a coral loveseat. I had to close the screen, take a sanity break, and start over. But in general, like Lean Cuisine, Internet porn's a real time-saver! Super handy for those who need to shave a few minutes off their masturbation schedule, which—who am I kidding?—is not me. I should probably get a job.

Part of what had always bothered me about porn was that it seemed like a mens-only club. While I had access to this world like every other sexually active human with a laptop, I personally lacked the emotional permission to explore it. *That, and I was irrationally terrified by pop-ups of local singles wanting to show me their tits. Could they see my tits?* Anyway, the first few times I'd looked at porn, I hadn't seen anything that represented my tastes. With a little more delving, I found that Internet smut could appeal to me, provided I overlooked a few things: the settings, the men, the endless gratuitous penetration shots, the spray tans, the dialogue, and the facials. But that's just me. Some girls clearly love a gob of jizz in the tear duct. Nevertheless, there's a concrete reason why I, and some other women, may not feel our tastes are represented in porn. The reality has been that men create mainstream porn for the pleasure of other men.

Here are a few generalizations about what mainstream hetero porn includes: women are always ready and waiting for sex; all women love anal; all women are up for getting it on with another woman (while, of course, men with other men is homosexual); women scream ecstatically when they orgasm (and always do); men always pull out to ejaculate (which, as all the girls on *16 and Pregnant* will attest, is patently untrue).

The fact that most porn is a male-oriented fantasy does not mean that women don't enjoy these things or have any of these desires too.

Contrary to what the Lifetime network would have us believe, we don't all want roses, candlelight, and sex in front of a roaring fireplace. Or maybe we want the bear rug one day and an anonymous quickie in an alleyway the next. The point is, when it comes to sex and porn, there is no one-size-fits-all. While a growing number of women watch porn, as with Hollywood movies, they still only produce a small percentage of it. Remember what a big deal it was when Kathryn Bigelow won the Oscar for best director? Or what a hoopla it was that *Bridesmaids* was a smart, funny film written by chicks? In porn, without deliberately looking for it, we don't see or know what a female perspective is. Things may be changing. But for the moment, it's still marginal.

While female porn viewership is growing, many women still feel uncomfortable with the topic. Maybe because, like me, you grew up with women's studies teachers in purple crushed-velvet dresses railing against female sexual subjugation. Or maybe you identify with feeling subtly betrayed by the thought of your guy getting off to his favorite pubeless, D-cup, cellulite-free Internet galpal when he could be rolling with your hot ass. Or maybe, like yours truly, you've never been afraid that if you vocally critiqued aspects of porn, you'd be labeled a ball-busting uptight prude. After all, feminism is *so out* this millennium.

For years, I didn't give porn the time of day because I assumed it wasn't for my pleasure. I dismissed the whole lot of it. Shaft, porn! I didn't search out other types of XXX than what was first spit out by the Internet, because the whole experience felt too uncomfortable. I felt that hard-core Internet porn should come with not only a "Must Be Over 18" warning but also "Beware of Massive Cocks!" I was a-okay with my battery-operated friend and my Channing fantasies. *Especially after I stood next to him in the security line at LAX. Heavens to Betsy.* Still, it was beginning to dawn on me that I might be missing out on something. That it was actually a shaft on *me,* not porn. Not because porn could necessarily make my life so much better. But because I believe that women engaging in discussions about XXX, and influencing the production of it, could make a better product. Heck, anything's possible, ladies, maybe even a better world.

It turns out that fall in LA is a lot like summer. In fact, it's even hotter. A colony of ants has sprung up in my kitchen with the extreme heat, and I battle not to leave an errant crumb. This isn't exactly easy, considering that I live with two men who breeze through the house discarding take-out containers. At the moment, there are often three dudes coming and going, as another one of Robbie's friends, Tom, has joined the show as a production assistant. At the moment, they are all in the living room packing up gear to leave. When I ask Tom how he likes it, he looks wide-eyed.

"A porn star was hitting on him yesterday," Robbie explains, patting Tom on the back.

"Lucky you," I say. "Did you get her number?"

"I don't think she's date material," he says.

"Right." How typical—the girls you jerk off to and the ones you date are different, I think, but I don't say anything. "So you'll call me if it's cool for me to come by?" I direct to Robbie instead.

"Yeah, absolutely. But don't get your hopes up, okay? We just never know how the day's going to evolve."

"I get it. Let me know," I say. Michel has told Robbie that when there's an appropriate moment, he'll ask if I can come on set. So I am on porn standby, awaiting my official invitation with bated breath.

I actually have focus groups to transcribe, so when the boys leave, I get to work. Hours pass with my headphones on, parsing together relevant quotes. I take a lunch break and make myself a turkey sandwich. Then I scrub the kitchen tiles spotless, squashing ants in my wake.

Around two o'clock Robbie calls and tells me that there's a good chance that I can come to the set in an hour or two. The location is a house in the Valley. Another poolside orgy scene. I hang up and shower so that I'm ready to go. I blow-dry my hair straight for good measure. What does one wear to a porn set? I choose skinny jeans, a tank top, and flip-flops. I will go as myself. As I put on mascara and blush in the mirror, I start to feel a bit nervous. Am I ready for this? Will it quell my wild imagination or make things worse? With the exception of Nine's gonzo debacle, Robbie generally reports that most shoots are businesslike and professional. I'm sure that will be good to see firsthand.

Ready to go at an instant, I continue my work. An hour passes, then two. Three. I make coffee. Bite my nails. Reapply lip gloss. I text Robbie, "what's up?" but get no response. At 6:00 PM he calls.

"Hey, I'm so sorry. I had to keep rolling and things are now winding down, so Michel says it would be best to postpone this. That okay?"

"Yeah, sure."

"We have to go do some establishing shots after this, so the boys and I will grab dinner. See you after."

We hang up and I slump back in my desk chair. As well as disappointed, I feel slightly relieved. I go to the bedroom and replace my outfit with leggings and a ratty sweatshirt. Then I grab a half-drunk bottle of white wine from the fridge and pour myself a glass. Hell, I'm not driving anywhere. I settle in on the couch for an evening of HBO.

In the next week I repeat this standby scenario two more times. I no longer bother getting primped. It's a frustrating situation, but I understand that Robbie can't snap his fingers and make it work out. He explains that it's delicate—Michel has to ask the performers' permission, and as a reality show they are already intruders on the regular flow of things. I am patient. I do my work. I pitch a story to *GQ* magazine and the editor actually responds! He says no, but whatever, I'm just deluded enough to find being rejected by a premier men's magazine encouraging. He says: "Best of luck. You might have better luck with the ladies' mags."

I plan to whip up a few more pitches. Instead, I watch more porn. I've discovered the "amateur category." And while I suspect that these naked Cirque du Soleil routines are not actually being performed by amateurs, the scenes are more my type of hot. Some of these people even look like they *want* to fuck each other! My new hobby has me walking around as damp in the culottes as a tween girl at a Bieber concert. Is this how Robbie always feels? Unfortunately, we never seem to have a moment alone these days. Matt and Tom are always around, shooting the shit, drinking beers on the lawn, going quiet when I come around. I feel constantly excluded from the boy's X-rated club. I try to chime in on their conversations—"How was the Valley today? Did you boys film some sweet ass?" They smile awkwardly. I serve them my Cindy Crawford strawberry-rhubarb pies, which they gobble up, say "Thanks, Em!" and then dump the sticky plates in the sink.

I meet Hilary in West Hollywood one day after her facial appointment and we peruse the wedding dresses at Monique Lhuillier. They are gorgeous and totally unattainable. We grab iced coffee, walk down Melrose, and stop in at Kiki de Montparnasse, a high-end lingerie store and sex boutique. I tell her all about the trials and tribulations of trying to get on a porn set. She sympathizes. We both try on ridiculously expensive lingerie. In the dressing rooms, they have Sergio Rossi high heels to model with our bustiers and camisoles. The lighting is flattering and there are plush chairs to relax on. Hot sales girls give us champagne to drink while we show off our looks to each other. We giggle and strut our stuff. I buy a lacy thong and novelty whip, which is all I can afford. Hilary buys a silk kimono. We both decide that more porn should happen in this environment, in this wardrobe. With that in mind, I decide that maybe executive producing my own pornographic experience is the way to go. At least in the comfort of my own home.

Later that night, I'm freshly waxed, sporting my new thong, drug-store thigh-highs, and stiletto heels. A bottle of Jack Daniel's, two shot glasses, my novelty whip, and a camera are on the coffee table in front of me. It is ten o'clock, and Robbie was supposed to be home an hour ago. Matt is away for a couple of nights in Montreal. Robbie is shooting with Tom and Michel. Since this is supposed to be a pleasant surprise, I don't want to bother him with "where the eff are you" texts. I pour a shot for myself and sip it. On the first night that Robbie and I hooked up we drank JD. This is my stab at naughty-meets-nostalgic.

Sometime around eleven, I hear the key in the door. I jump up from my slumped position where I've been reading *Elle*, toss my hair, and attempt to look casually sexy.

"Hey," he says, coming through the door, heaving bags into the entryway. Followed by "Well, hello there. What's all this?"

"Just waiting for my man to come home," I say.

"Wow, you look hot." He walks in front of the television, facing me.

"Whiskey after a hard day, my love?"

"Sure," he says. "Just let me go to the bathroom." He walks to the other room. I listen to him pee with the door open, behavior that we're both guilty of, but that doesn't really stoke my libido. He blows his nose and comes back, sits on the corner of the couch and takes his sweaty work boots off, then shuffles back along the sectional, reclining his head onto my lap.

"Hi," he says.

"Hi, long day?"

"Yeah, just give me a minute and then I'll take advantage of you."

"I'll happily take advantage of you," I say.

"*Mmm*," he says and closes his eyes. I'm still for a minute. Worried that this will be the end of my much-anticipated plan, I shimmy out from under him and replace my legs with a pillow. Then I set to work undressing him. He lets out a few encouraging moans. I take it as incentive to go down on him. As I pull down his boxers, I am met with the full-force pungency of a man who has been working in the heat all day. Christ, a little *cologne d'homme* is a turn-on for me, but this shit is noxious. It doesn't help that he hasn't had a trim down here in, what, five months? But I am determined. I hold my breath and open wide. Things get going. Until I need to breathe. In a moment of genius, I stand up and bend over the coffee table—a position I know he'll appreciate in my thigh highs and heels. Phew, saved.

"You're so hot." He sits up on the couch and goes down on me from behind, sliding my G-string out of the way. I moan—louder and more enthusiastically than I ever used to, thanks to my recent porn reeducation.

"*Mmm*, yeah, baby," he says, clearly digging the new, unleashed me. He stands and wraps his fingers around the front of my hips, bends his knees to fit into the backs of mine (I'm a good eight inches shorter than he, even in stilettos), and penetrates me. This is hot. I'm feeling downright pleased with myself. I continue to shout encouragement: "*Yeah, yeah, yeah!*" When out of nowhere Robbie rams me so hard that I fly off of him and land on the coffee table, ass up. I smack the bottle of Jack with my forearm, and the bottle skids and crashes to the floor.

"What the fuck?!!!" I scream.

"My leg, my leg, it's cramping!" Robbie yells, falling backward onto the couch, not helping me. I peel myself off the coffee table and pick up the Jack, miraculously unbroken. Robbie clutches his thigh in pain and writhes back and forth.

"Are you okay?"

"This is crazy," he winces. "Can you rub it?"

I shimmy a corner of my bare ass onto the only free space on the couch and knead his thigh with my thumbs.

"Ouch, watch the leg hair!" he says.

You're kidding me, jackass. Instead, I give a motherly "Shhh, it will pass." In a moment or two he relaxes and becomes aware of me again.

"Are you okay?" he asks.

"I may not bear children," I answer.

"I'm so sorry, come here," he says, extending his arms. I lie on top of him. We hug. I bury my face in his neck. "Mmm," he says. His breathing slows. Is he falling asleep?

"We're not done here," I say, lifting my head.

"Hmmm?" he says.

No way is this the end of my hot night in. I sit up, straddling him, and bring both of his hands onto my tits, still plumped by underwire and encased in black lace. He smiles. I move my hips atop his and look down to assess the situation. *We are not in business.* I continue my grinding, jerk him to half-mast, and then attempt to stuff him into my cha cha. His dick slinks out of me like cooked tagliatelle.

"Hey," he says and makes eye contact with me—as focused as Serena Williams. "I want to be into this but I'm exhausted. Let's try again later? Don't be offended. Are you hungry?"

I am, in fact, starved. I don't want him to see the full force of my disappointment or what a pathetically big deal this was for me. So I climb off, turn, and walk toward the bedroom. "Sure. Let's order pizza. I'm going to change. I'll have a slice of whatever you want and get me a side Caesar salad, please. And a Diet Coke."

"Okay. Em?"

"Yeah?"

"I love that you did this for me."

"Anytime," I lie. I go to the bedroom and hastily pull off my thigh-highs, ripping them in the process and thinking, *Robbie was supposed to do that.* I replace my uncomfortable bra and thong with full-coverage panties up to my belly button and my old, worn, baby-blue sweats, size large. Fuck all this fucking shit. I yank on a tank top and regard my smoky eye makeup in the mirror. I went all out, tried to get all Eva Angelina, and look what happened? We are *so not* trying again later. I want to cry. Maybe I'll be able to laugh tomorrow. For now, I wipe off my mascara, liquid liner, and sparkly plum eye shadow, and toss the smeared tissues in the trash.

A week later we're at a random barbecue in the Hollywood hills. This Parisian guy, Jean Luc, who's a friend of a friend, invited us. I'm not crazy about him. He's arrogant. But he always knows where the party is. Robbie, Matt, Tom, Hilary and her boyfriend Tucker, and a few others are here. We're in the backyard overlooking LA's sprawling lights. People are grilling things, drinking. I tell Hilary about my botched sexcapade and she laughs.

"So you just ordered pizza?"

"Yeah, and watched fucking *Notting Hill* on TV—again."

"That's pretty bad."

"The worst."

"But it's also super normal. Tucker and I sleep on the couch in front of the TV these days more than we make it into bed. And we're having sex a bit less since living together. You guys?"

"Yeah, when I arrived it was every day, now it's every couple of days. It's hard not to see it as a measure of our relationship. Here I am trying to keep up with the girls he sees at work, and he just wants to scratch his ass and eat mac and cheese when he gets home."

"Typical."

"Ugh, we're a bad married-people sitcom already."

"I think it actually does happen to all of us," she says and then nods to our empty glasses. "We need more champagne."

The night evolves into a dance party. People get in the hot tub. Sprawl out smoking on the lawn. Dance more on the terrace. Around 3:00 AM, Robbie and I decide to make our exit.

"Thanks for inviting us, buddy," Robbie says to Jean Luc, who is standing with his arm draped over my shoulder in a creepy way. He leans in and gives me two almost-on-the-mouth kisses.

"Hey, you and your bee-uutiful fiancé are always welcome," he croons. "Especially after having me come by set last week."

I stare at them.

"You went to see them filming *Webdreams*?" I say, incredulous.

"Yeah, so cool buddy. So cool," he says.

We step out onto the porch and walk down the street to our car. I walk ahead of Robbie.

"Em, Matt called Jean Luc and he came by. I had nothing to do with it," he says.

"Right," I say.

"Michel wasn't even there. Matt would be in big shit if he knew about it."

"Okay! Whatever!!" I yell over Hollywood.

"Hey, come on. What's the big deal?" I turn on my heels to face him.

"The big deal is that I've been trying to come see what you do *every day*, and I've been having trouble with this scenario from day one, and working my ass off *not* to, and getting Brazilians and wearing fucking skanky lingerie and that arrogant French dick-fuck gets to go to set just because he's a guy and it's *so cool* to see porn in action?! Why didn't Matt call *me*? Why didn't you tell me? What about my article? Does it mean nothing to you that I'm trying to land paid writing work? Why am I always the fucking leper?" I picture my palm meeting Robbie's cheekbone, imagine his head spin with the impact. I clench my right fist. My eyes burn with the violent image. I stand perfectly still, my fury paralyzing me like Novocain. One move is all it will take to do something irreversible.

Robbie doesn't respond. He stands, stunned, holding the car keys, then slowly walks to the passenger's side door and opens it for me. I climb in, all sharp, controlled movements. Buckle up. Seethe. *Fucking boys' club.*

We drive home in silence.

CHAPTER 9

FANTASY

"Are you going to talk to me now?" Robbie says the next morning. Last night we drove through the shadowy Hollywood hills in silence. Went to bed without a word. We've now both awoken and showered in silence. I sport a towel on my head. The fascist sun streams through the window as I pull on pink underwear covered in galloping horses and an ancient, flesh-colored bra. *How about a little rain, LA? Some darkening clouds in the distance, perchance? Do you ever give your citizens permission to loaf and be miserable?* Not today, apparently. I zip up jeans; don a tank top, cardigan, and flip-flops—the usual. I run a brush through my wet, tangled hair and apply mascara, all the while watching Robbie in the bedroom mirror. He pulls on a clean t-shirt and stuffs his old Red Sox sleep shirt under the pillow.

"I had nothing to do with Jean Luc coming to set," he says. "It was all Matt. I didn't expect to see him there. He didn't run it by me or Michel."

My mascara is goopy, and who knows how old; it's time to spend $6.99 on a new hot-pink tube. I separate lashes with my index fingernail. Twist the nasty, smeared cap back on. I busy myself by rummaging through my leopard-print jewelry box for nothing in particular, forcibly ignoring Rob.

"Em? You're killing me," he comes up behind me. We make stoic eye contact in the mirror.

"How many of your friends have you hired on this show now? Let's see: there's Matt—oh, and John, who worked for a few days until he decided he didn't want his Catholic relatives finding out—then Tom, Jamie, George. Am I forgetting anyone? Oh, Jean Luc—my bad. Lucky six!"

"Everyone but Jean Luc *worked* on the show. They didn't just come by to check out porn stars. Most of my friends here are from film school. We always help each other get work. That's how it goes. You know that."

"Sure, whatever." I turn to walk away but he grabs my arm.

"What, you don't believe me?" I shrug off his hold and leave the bedroom. He follows me to the kitchen. "This is ridiculous," he says. "You can't be mad at me for this. This is not my fault."

I open the fridge and survey the contents: lemons, beer, radishes, Tropicana, not much else. I grab the box of juice and take a glass from the cupboard. I pour some for myself.

"I'll have some too, please," Robbie says. I smack another glass on the white-tiled counter in front of him, along with the juice, and turn to leave. "I wasn't going to tell you this now, but Michel said he doesn't think you can come by set after all, ever. It's not going to happen."

"What?" I stop in the doorframe and turn to face Robbie.

"We're behind schedule, Production is pissed, and when I asked him again the other day, he basically got irritated and told me no."

"Wow. So that's it, huh? No fighting for me?"

"I'm not going to jeopardize my job over this!"

"That's a bit dramatic," I say.

"I'm dramatic? Really?"

I spin on my heels, sending a spray of OJ droplets across the dining room floor. I return to our room and shimmy back under the duvet in my clothes. A few minutes later, I hear Robbie and Matt leave the house, off to the porn world. I don't bother to get up for several hours. I close my eyes to block out the sun; my inner world burns orange. I wait for my anger and frustration to seep out of me. Eventually it dissipates, or at least displaces, storing up somewhere else—like my kidneys or maybe the box spring.

When he comes home that night, we don't discuss our argument further. Days pass. We gradually soften around each other without ever verbally making up. I've silently chosen to give up addressing *Webdreams* altogether with Rob—no more porn talk whatsoever. Take that! As you can imagine, Robbie is taking it quite well, taking it like a Bermuda fucking vacation, like an icy-cold summer ale.

The next week, I'm in the apartment upstairs from ours attempting to take down a filthy venetian blind twice the length of me. I've managed to unhinge the thing from its bracket; it sways back and forth like a teeter-totter. Years' worth of dust settles across my t-shirt and invades my nasal passageways. I stagger awkwardly to the apartment door and begin my descent to the courtyard, where the plan is to somehow mount this fucker on the clothesline and hose it down. Initially, this seemed easier than washing each plastic slat individually, which in my approximation would have taken twenty-four hours. On second consideration, my alternate approach is also flawed. It smacks back and forth on either side of the wall as I maneuver down the narrow staircase. It'd better not break.

Why am I performing this ridiculous circus act? As of recently, Robbie and I hold the proud title of Apartment Managers. The previous apartment manager tragically died of cancer a few months ago. Seeing an opportunity to save on rent, Robbie waited a tactful amount of time, and then pitched our landlord, Victor, on us as a management duo. Between Rob's handyman skills and the fact that I rarely leave the house, we were a shoo-in. The job is now ours. I figured I could fulfill the more glamorous role of answering phone calls from tenants and calling plumbers. Now, of course, Rob's away just when the upstairs apartment needs to be cleaned and fixed up for new tenants. Where's my darling? He's in Vegas filming the AVN Awards—the Oscars of porn—where they give out medals for categories like best girl-on-girl, best blowjob, what have you.

I'm dueling with a blind and a garden hose. This is just the beginning. There are at least five more wretched venetians in the apartment and I'm already sweating profusely. I can tell by the tenant who just walked past me with averted eyes that I look certifiable in my '70s running shorts, smeared white t-shirt, and a bandana holding back my tangle of hair.

I somehow manage to hoist the thing and hose it down while only bending two of the slats irreversibly. Clean and slightly damaged is better than revolting though, right? I hope Victor, our landlord, thinks so. I leave the blind hanging to dry and carry the next one downstairs. By number three, I'm getting pretty good at this pony trick. It isn't so bad. It's officially winter and the weather is really quite glorious. The courtyard fountain bubbles; the pink and red roses perpetually bloom. The sky overhead is robin's-egg blue. Things could be worse.

Twenty minutes later, I want to kill myself. Having completed hosing the venetians and moved on to repainting over plastered holes while the blinds dry, I manage to coat my hands and arms up to my elbows in non-water-soluble paint. With a piece of plastic over my paint-dipped index finger, I dial Robbie's number on speaker.

"How do you get oil-based paint off?" I yell at the phone.

"What? Where are you?" he says.

"Upstairs! Renovating, fuck!"

"You'll need paint thinner," he says. "There should be some in the supply closet. We're rolling, can I call you back?"

"Yup," I hang up the phone. I wonder whom or what he's filming. I have an idea from Googling the AVN Awards website—tits and ass sheathed in lace and leather. Girls smiling with heads cocked, tongues licking teeth suggestively. I cover my hands in grocery-bag bondage and descend to the supply closet. Landlord Victor is here. He is tall, tanned, and forever clad like a Floridian—white sneakers, tan shorts, Hawaiian shirt.

"Oh, hi," I say.

"I see you're cleaning the blinds," he says. "Don't leave them out there long."

"Yup, spiffing them up!" I say faux-joyfully. "I'm just about to bring them in." We both look at my hands covered in paint and plastic bags. It's obvious that I'm not just about to do anything. "Any paint thinner in there?"

Victor is a man of few words. He hands me a can and I scamper off before he has a chance to ask me any other questions, which proves how patently unfit for the job I am. I sponge-bathe myself in toxic liquid, remount the blinds, and decide to call it a day.

Sewage-colored water runs off me in the shower. I shampoo twice, towel off, and crack a beer on the couch. I look around our messy apartment—how the hell did it get like this? Not the mess, but my life, the constant solitude. The steps are easy enough to trace back—falling in love in Montreal, two years in grad school and a long-distance relationship, a proposal, a move to LA, a fiancé who's always at work filming money shots, me freelancing from home. Robbie always says that he would follow me somewhere if the roles were reversed. But they're not, and I can't foresee them ever being so. Which means I'm the follower. I am home alone, yet again, with none of the drama or intrigue of the motion picture by the same name. Sometimes I feel like I have spent the majority of my life alone and that I'm destined to pass my waking hours with just my dribbling thoughts as company. My days already bear a disturbingly strong resemblance to my grandmother's days in her geriatric home, only with less bingo. Man, I wish someone would come over and play bingo with me.

Now, I realize that *being with oneself* is more or less the human condition. But my lifestyle choices always seem to push aloneness to the extreme. Do I ask for this? Maybe. In elementary and high school I used to exaggerate sickness in order to have a day by myself with the company of soap operas and McCain oven fries. My mom indulged this impulse and would allow me a certain number of what we dubbed "mental health days." I appreciated, and still appreciate, her take on the matter. We Southwoods are a private and reclusive people. Of course, to top it off, I've aspired to be a writer, otherwise known as a crazy, depressive loner. I have to heave myself out into the world, earn my mental health benefits by having *some* interaction with the human race.

Alas, I've already learned this lesson. Once, in my midtwenties, sick of bartending, boyfriends, and city life, I booked a flight to Spain to "get away from it all." This rationale elicited an understanding nod from my peers, as if I were fleeing persecution, not middle-class existential angst. Thus, I travelled alone to a remote northern Spanish town and paid up-front to rent a small house for a month. It was only when I shut the door to my haunted casita in utter solitude that I realized my version of "getting away" brought me uncomfortably close to myself. It was like an ashram minus the ashram. I did not have a transcendent experience. I did not learn to eat, pray, or love. I read the only book I'd brought—*The Famished Road*—thrice (which, as indicated by the title, isn't a particularly uplifting read), watched *The Gilmore Girls* in Spanish nightly while eating my weight in European-style vanilla yogurt, and consequently picked up jogging up hillsides like a lame mountain goat in the uncomfortable hiking boots I'd brought. I made no friends. It was the longest thirty days of my life.

I hear most twenty-four-year-olds do not experience Europe this way. They buy rail passes. Stay in hostels with raucous Brits. Throw up in fountains. Sleep with randoms. Not me!

The dance usually goes something like this: When surrounded by people as I was last summer in Canada—relatives hovering everywhere wanting to make day plans, cold-cut lunches, and incessant chatter—I desperately want to retreat. Now here, alone, day after day, I want to be distracted from myself and I need humans and/or alcohol to do that. I gravitate to extremes but finding moderation in all things might help prevent me from a stay at the Betty Ford Clinic.

I call Hilary. She says there's a party in the hills somewhere. Twenty minutes later we're zipping up there in the Mini Cooper she's leased because the Merc finally died with a thud in a downtown parking lot. Now we are speedy. On the way, we pick up her hipster friend whose name sounds like Alaska through the Clap Your Hands Say Yeah song that's blaring. Alaska is wearing some sort of belted poncho, sunglasses at night, and ankle boots. I am wearing black jeans, pumps, and a button-down, which suddenly has me feeling very business casual. We wind our way up narrow streets in a direction I could never retrace. The road is only wide enough for one car. I'm glad I'm not driving. I'm glad we're in a Mini. We park between two enormous SUVs at a forty-five-degree angle and tumble out onto the curb.

Hil reads out the address from her phone as we walk. Soon the thump of bass and sidewalk lingerers make it redundant. We make our way through a gate between two high brick walls, and then pass through the open door into the house. An art-lined hallway leads into a stainless-steel kitchen where people stand elbow to elbow. I grab a beer from a pail of ice. Hilary and Alaska make cocktails on a counter that's littered with giant drugstore bottles of vodka, rum, and mixers. I take a solo stroll to survey the scene. The living room is a dance party. Modern grey couches are pushed to the side. Lights flash in rhythm to the music. Hipsters trip out to techno. I'm not drunk enough for such shenanigans. I sidle my way between partygoers out to the balcony, which extends along the back of the house. We overhang a haze of smoggy, twinkling lights—the quintessential LA view, I'm learning. Is that downtown in the distance or Century City? I have no idea which direction we're facing. It's smoky out here, loud with chatter. I weave my way back into the kitchen, but Hil is gone. I see Alaska sitting on someone's lap by the dance floor. I scan the room but don't see Hilary. It's so crowded that it takes me a minute to realize there's a guy, exactly my height, standing right in front of me. Our noses are only a few inches apart. I crack up.

"Looking for someone?" he says.

"Yeah, my friends," I yell.

"Good luck with that."

"Right, thanks." I can barely hear him over the music. I move over to let people pass by and wind up along the kitchen wall. Dude follows. We get to chatting. He asks me what I do. Half seriously, I say I'm a poet. He says he's a poet too. I tell him I'm from Montreal. He's from New York.

We have the same East-versus-West conversation I've now had one zillion times—the weather, the lack of walking in LA. We discuss our favorite poets. His is Frank O'Hara. Mine, Anne Carson. He asks for my phone number and I tell him I'm engaged to be married but in need of friends. He says we should have tea sometime. I say okay, give him my digits. I go on another hunt for Hilary, starting with the balcony. She's here smoking, gesticulating.

"There you are!" she says.

"I made a friend," I say.

"Look at you!"

"I know, impressive. He's over there." I point him out through the window inside. He's now standing on the periphery of people dancing.

"He looks like a troll," she says. He does, in fact, kind of have a gnome thing going on, but I think that might be a good thing in a guy friend.

I get home around two in the morning and call Robbie. We're both tipsy. He says he's been at some kind of after-party in the Hugh Hefner suite, but that it wasn't anything like it sounds—libidinous, illicit. There were more tech geeks than porn stars, blah, blah, blah. *Oh shut up, stick a dildo in it,* I think. I don't even want to know how his night was. He tells me I sound far away. I say I'm tired. We hang up, and I sleep on the couch in my casual Friday's outfit, with an open bag of chips on my stomach.

Not caring used to come more easily to me. Back when Robbie and I first started dating, I teetered blissfully on the edge of indifference; I acted infuriatingly blasé. He once said to me, "I wonder if this would be easier if I had your heart?" I think I shrugged at the time. He was right, he confirmed to me recently: now that he has my heart, it's easier for him. He feels cozy and secure in love. Snug as a bug. But when *I'm* chin-deep in a relationship, I feel the opposite of comfy, unable to find the steady poise between emotionally distant and psychotically attached. It feels dangerous to care so much. Is it completely insane that I am about to get married and still wondering how people do this love dance and not get eaten alive or wind up eating off their own hands?

Oh, I don't mean to be so dramatic. I'm not a teenager in hapless, consuming love; I'm a nearly thirty-year-old engaged woman! I'm a totally pulled-together chick who only occasionally sleeps on the couch cuddling a bag of Ruffles. In theory, I comprehend the notion of letting there be space between two people. I've read that Kahlil Gibran fellow. I know, intellectually, that two separate whole beings with the breeze blowing between them make the best match. Still, I constantly forget how to live this out practically. *Especially these days.* I find myself wanting to be either composite metal or oceans apart. So right now, tranquilizing my emotions and staying distant from Robbie's reality feels the safest. Which begs the question, am I making a huge mistake delving into something I'm not ready for? Not nearly mature enough for now, or possibly ever, given my apparent emotional maturity level: thirteen-and-a-half?

The troll calls me the next day. We make a date to meet that evening at a Moroccan teahouse in Silver Lake. He's sitting at a table by the window when I arrive at five. The sky is dark already; the air is chilly. Inside it's cozy, smells nutty and a little floral. Customers work on laptops or chat tête-à-tête over teapots. We order a pot of rooibos tea to share. He tells me about his divorce. He moved to LA recently from New York to escape the wreckage. Packed up a van full of belongings and hit the road.

"A lot of people my age are getting divorced," he says. His age is my age. I, too, know a few couples that jumped in early and are already bailing out. We dub it "the tragedy of the twentysomething marriages." I tell him I'm on the opposite side of the fence—pumped, nearly thirty, ready to go! I tell him about Robbie's job like it's no big deal to me, which is how I always tell people about it. I certainly don't say that my guy filming pornography has me acting jealous, skeptical of the human race, and certifiably insane. *That's clearly way too much info for a casual guy pal.*

He asks me if I want to go see some live music in Laurel Canyon. He's writing an article about this group of musicians that get together and jam. I say sure. We get into his divorce getaway van and drive up into the hills.

The venue is at someone's house that doubles as a recording studio, and I feel like I've walked right into the '70s. Tapestries hang from the walls. Guitars, drum kits, and random ukuleles abound. We walk through the kitchen to the back patio where benches with macramé pillows invite you to lie down, drop acid, and stare at the LA smog. The troll introduces me around to various lanky, bell-bottom-clad men, including Chris Robinson from the band The Black Crowes. I think my knees might give out. I have always had a weird celebrity crush on him, or more precisely, on him and Kate Hudson together. They are my hippy-slash-Hollywood daydream power couple, or at least they were until they divorced. He flips his hair back and says "Hey" to me. Those straggly locks settling on the shoulder of that lanky man are not every girl's fantasy. But they're mine. *Lord have mercy.*

The night evolves into an endless jam session seen through a haze of narcotic smoke. The troll is attentive to me. He brings me cold beers and occasionally hands me a bottle of whiskey to swig on. I sway to the tunes. People stand up to strum or sing and then bow out. A few dudes who are easily in their sixties breeze through at one point. I'm pretty sure they are famous from the reaction they receive, but I don't know who they are. Maybe they're the Allman Brothers? The Band? Who the fuck knows? Who cares—I love everyone. Twin girls with deep southern accents join them to belt out a soulful ballad.

I'm having an amazing time. I adore nights like this that come out of nowhere and take you to another world. I feel free, and blessed, and yes, sufficiently high on substances and atmosphere. Without noticing the passage of time, I realize that it's four in the morning. The troll asks me if I want to leave. I shrug. We stay another hour sitting out on the back patio listening to my new friend Chris tell stories about his adorable son Ryder. I gape like a groupie and make the occasional comment much, much too loud. The troll offers me more whiskey, a blanket for my shoulders. I accept both.

By the time we pull up in front of my apartment, the sun is coming up. I wonder if I will sleep or just curl up on the couch and read or write a poem—I often have this idiotic delusion at dawn knowing full well that poems are better composed on eight hours of sleep and stiff coffee. I thank my new friend for the adventure. He says it was his pleasure and leans in to kiss me. I lurch backward toward the passenger-side window and hit my head.

He retreats. I look at him, the scenario, the rising sunshine. Shit. Does he think I led him on? Staying out all night, acting, for all appearances, single and free-loving? "I'm going to go," I say. "Good night. Good morning. Bye."

I shut the van door with a tinny thud. He pulls away. Inside, sun is beginning to light up the living room. I pull off my boots and jeans, now sporting just a slouchy sweater. I put on water to boil for tea and survey the contents of the cupboard. The last exchange I had with Robbie was a text that said "at a party, call you soon!" But I never did. He's probably sleeping now, the sun filtering through his blinds in a Vegas hotel room. I wish he were here to climb in bed with. I grab a chocolate cookie with my chamomile and go to the bedroom. I slide into the cool sheets, feeling far from Robbie, and fall asleep before drinking my tea.

I wake a few hours later and call Hilary. She doesn't think I should tell Robbie about the troll's pass at me. I think she's probably right. I don't want him feeling suspicious and untrusting of me having male friends. It's been hard enough to make pals in this city. I'll just have to relegate any guy friendships to group settings, daylight hours, sobriety. Hil tells me about a married man she became friends with when she first moved here who tried to take it to the next level. We both agree that, if we are honest with ourselves, we sensed their intentions. The attention feels nice until shit gets real. I know that I was using the troll's interest as a respite from the insecurity and turmoil I've been feeling with Robbie. But I don't want to be the messy girl with murky boundaries that I was five years ago. She was a hot mess.

I speak to Robbie midmorning.

"You never called," he says.

"I'm so sorry, the night got away from me. I didn't mean to make you worry."

"Is everything okay?"

"Yes, I had a fun night at this party in Laurel Canyon and before I knew it, it was morning."

"Should I be concerned?"

"No," I say.

"How's your new friend?"

"He's fine. He brought me home safely," I say, which is the better part of the truth. Robbie tells me he has to get to work. We hang up. I feel like shit. I sleep for another hour and then return to fixing the upstairs apartment in another tragic outfit.

The next night, I am still doing penance. The apartment is spotless and I am sober, alone, watching a three-hour commercial version of *Sweet*

Home Alabama on the couch. Robbie comes home tomorrow. He texts me to say they are going out to celebrate their last night in Vegas. I say "have fun, call and say goodnight." I make popcorn and pass time in romantic comedy la-la land. The movie climaxes when Reese Witherspoon leaves Patrick Dempsey at the altar. Robbie texts me a picture of himself. He's holding a beer in a rooftop hot tub perched over Sin City. "Miss you!!!" the caption says. I'm sure he means it genuinely, but at the moment it comes off as mocking. *Sure, as if you miss me from the Vegas rooftop party, jackass.* I start to cry. I miss him terribly. Not just since he's been away, but also because I've felt so far from him these last months, at a time when we're supposed to be the closest. Our wedding invitations are on the dining room table. They've been there for months because we can't seem to get around to them. We've been avoiding finalizing the guest list because we can't agree on who makes the final cut. Shit's a mess. I want to call him and unload, but I don't even know what I'd say. Besides, it's so not the time. I won't interrupt his night out just because I'm still recovering from the emotional hangover of mine. I let my tears roll down my cheeks and shove popcorn in my mouth as I watch Reese choose the man she's supposed to be with, the one who's been there all along. Comedic relief follows catharsis. Credits roll. I run myself a bath, climb in, and cover my now-puffy face with a warm washcloth. I am such an unbelievable sap.

I'm asleep in bed a few hours later when a text wakes me. Except it's not a text, it's junk email telling me how to meet LA singles. I left the sound on in case Robbie called. It's four in the morning and he hasn't. I text "you still out?" And lie there waiting for a reply. I think about calling but I don't really want to be that girl right now. Is this punishment for the other night? Tit for tat? I listen to helicopters circling over Hollywood. Dogs bark. I drift into a half sleep but keep waking on the hour: 5:00 AM,

6:00 AM, still nothing. Eventually I pass out and wake at 9:30. I call his phone and it goes straight to voicemail.

"Hi, I'm worried. Please call me," I say. Then hang up. Panic rises within me. I get up out of bed. Make coffee. Call Matt.

"I don't mean to bug you, but I'm looking for Robbie and his phone is off. Do you know where he is?"

"Shit, Em. I don't. We've been looking for him too. We're supposed to drive back to LA in an hour. Don't panic. I'll call you back soon."

I look down at the phone and mentally go through the options. Best scenario: maybe he passed out dead drunk, forgot to charge his phone, and is still asleep. However, there is the possibility that he left it in a cab or it slid out of his pocket while he was getting a lap dance. He may be on a Hunter S. Thompson trip in the desert somewhere making angels in the sand. Or perhaps he's left me for another woman and downing a midmorning scotch while figuring out how to tell me. I turn on the TV to kill time. Patrick Dempsey's dopey face stares back at me. *Sweet Home Alabama* is on again. You've got to be fucking kidding me.

At 11:30, the phone rings. It's Matt's number but Robbie's voice is on the other end of the line. He sounds like a rake across gravel.

"Hi. I blacked out last night at Brad's house and slept until now. I'm so sorry. I've never been so hungover in my life."

"I was really worried." A wave of emotions passes though me— relief, anger, suspicion. "What happened last night?"

"I met up with Brad at about 3:00 AM. We went to his restaurant to eat caviar and drink champagne in the storage room and then ended up back in the hot tub at his apartment with Crystal."

"Who's Crystal?" I say. I know Brad is an old friend of Rob's who manages hotels in Vegas. But I don't know anyone named goddamned *Crystal*.

"His girlfriend. I guess I passed out on their couch. I don't even remember. Matt just picked me up and I have to get my stuff from the hotel because we're driving back to LA now. I think I'm going to vomit. Can I call you in a bit?"

"Yeah, okay."

"I love you."

"I love you too," I say and hang up. Sucks to be retching your way back to LA, as countless souls can attest. Now that my panic has subsided, exhaustion takes its place. I guess we're both seeking a little escapism these days. I need normalcy, whatever that means. For now, I climb back into bed to try for another hour of sleep.

Later that night Robbie, Matt, and I are on the couch together eating Thai food. My Martha Stewart days are nowhere to be found. Robbie looks like I feel inside—wounded. He's been profusely apologetic since arriving home, and I don't care to punish him further. We've both been fuck-ups. Since Robbie is officially brain-dead, Matt gives me the rundown of the trip. He tells me that they never even got into the AVN Awards to film. They were denied at the door because they didn't have tickets and their filming status didn't hold the clout they'd hoped. They hoofed it to the Vegas porn convention instead, where they trailed the talent and interviewed the odd porn star. It wasn't great bang for their buck, so to speak.

"Sounds fun," I say. "Anyone want a beer?" Robbie looks at me dubiously; he's still green, poisoned. Matt says sure. I walk to the kitchen and grab two Tecates from the fridge. I'm sure the stuff Matt's saying about the show is true. But I still feel like I'm getting the wife's version of Vegas. *You know, the version that doesn't include strippers and prostitutes.* In another one of those couples honesty moments, Robbie once told me about an acquaintance of his who does an annual boys' trip to Vegas with a stash of Viagra. Why's that? Naturally, it's because the gang usually orders up a couple of prostitutes.

"You don't meet any girls when you go out with a bunch of dudes," Robbie's friend had told him. So they bring a couple of paid girls along to the club. Then, depending on what happens over the course of the night, everyone has someone to fuck. Or sometimes they just stay in their hotel suite and play Pass the Prostitute. I'd stared wide-eyed at Robbie. Okay, okay, I guess I tenuously knew this kind of thing happened—but that guy? Really? It was weird to put a face to such behavior—a strikingly handsome face, as it happens.

"I always figured girls would fall all over that guy," I'd said.

"I guess he just doesn't want the hassle," he'd said.

"Wow, yeah, I guess not." *Never trust the super-hot ones.*

I guess if Robbie were going to get up to such shenanigans, he'd probably be wise enough not to tell me stories like this about his friends. Then again, maybe he's extra calculated and plays the honesty card to throw me off the trail. I shake my head. What am I on about? *Just drink your watery Mexican beer, psychopath.*

I walk back into the living room and hand Matt a can. In the last thirty seconds, Robbie has passed out and now snores with his mouth gaping open. I sit on the couch between the boys and prop my feet on the coffee table. Prostitutes and strippers and porn stars, oh my! I slug my beer, gulp down the carbonation. Maybe the wife's version of Vegas is the one I want, given my recent brushes with the truth.

CHAPTER 10

SWALLOWING

I'm sick. Yesterday I woke up with stabbing pain in my throat. I tend toward throat infections. I spent a good part of my early twenties with various forms of tonsillitis, bronchitis, and strep throat; it was super fun. My mother's herbalist performs something called "body talk," wherein you lie on a massage table and she hovers over you, mumbling and lightly touching different body parts as she communes with your organs. Anyway, she was doing that to me once when she said "The throat is our communication center; we get infections when we're not expressing ourselves." At the time, I thought that might be a wee bit obvious for an organ whisperer. But I always think about it when I get sore throats. Is there something I'm not communicating? Whatever, my body aches. My head hurts. I can't think, let alone talk—no shit, I'm blocked. I exchange my pajamas for leggings, a turtleneck, and a wooly cardigan for my trip to the doctor. I've Googled a walk-in clinic that accepts my budget insurance plan. Robbie and Matt are filming at Rylie Spence's S&M loft in downtown LA. I have the car. I speed over in the Hyundai—and by "speed" I mean I drive twenty-five miles an hour and stall thrice.

The nice woman in blue scrubs at the clinic's registration counter patiently helps me fill out my forms, which I mess up several times even with direct supervision. At the moment I miss Canada, where you hand over your health card and you're good to go. No questions asked. Instead, I hand over my debit card and she dings me a hundred dollars. I sit deject-edly in the waiting area and watch the news on a small, wall-mounted TV. A toothy local reporter brandishes a microphone under a palm tree in the sun. I hate my life.

A nurse escorts me into the examination room, takes my vitals, and asks me to step on the scale. *Is this really necessary for assessing my throat infection?* I look at her sideways.

"I'll subtract two pounds for your clothes," she says, as if that's the usual concern. All tallied, I sit my butt down on the crinkly, paper-cov-ered exam table and await the doctor. I read the various signage in the room—disposal for medical waste, instructions for washing your hands. Five minutes later, the doctor shows up.

"How are we?" a slim, presumably gay, late-thirtysomething guy says. He looks up at me from his clipboard. "Oh, not so good. What can I do you for?"

"My throat hurts. I think it might be strep," I gurgle.

"Have you had it before?"

"Yes, many times," I reply. He gets out his throat culture kit and asks me to open wide. He makes a clucking noise and shakes his head.

"That looks like it hurts," he says.

"A wot," I say with the tongue depressor still in my mouth.

"Well, we're going to go ahead and start you on antibiotics," he says, scribbling on his prescription pad. "I'm also going to give you some Demerol for the pain. So tell work you're not coming in, go home, and space out on narcotics for a few days. Got it?"

I nod. I don't bother to tell him I'm unemployed, currently supported by my fiancé who's filming porn. But wait, did Doogie just tell me to go home and get high? I think he did. I no longer miss Canada. Back home, they don't prescribe the good drugs unless you drop several car batteries on your foot. I thank my dealer and head back out to the sunny parking lot. A quick stop at Rite Aid, and another small fortune later, I am home. Joyfully sedated, I watch *TLC* and drink Gatorade for ten hours.

Two days later, I feel marginally better and I need more sick-person supplies. Robbie is working, so I hoof it to the Ralphs around the corner. I hate Ralphs. First, there's the name. Is *ralph*—also the colloquialism "to puke"—really the best choice for a food store, folks? I'm not sure. Second, with a coat of paint and bright lights, they've clearly tried to elevate the perception of Ralphs from budget chains like Von's, while remaining a step below the wallet rape that is Whole Foods. Translation: The produce is below average but overly priced. Should lemons be $1.99 each in California? I don't believe so. Third, I see no logic behind the organization in here. Why is half the rice alongside the pasta while the other half is stuffed in the Latin-slash-Asian section? It's confusing. I always get lost. Today is no different—I'm on a maddening hunt for rice milk. It doesn't help that I'm stoned on Demerol.

I have walked all of the aisles no less than six times with my cumbersome basket full of canned soup when I finally remember that the rice milk is next to the cereal, not with all the other milk. But of course! I trudge over there and peruse the aisle, trying to scope out the familiar blue box. I can't see it. We've got Honey Bunches of Oats, All-Bran, various peanut and chocolate chip–laden cereal bars. I am swaying back and forth trying to focus when I spot it. I step in to grab a box. A small black-haired kid darts past at the same time, and we nearly smack foreheads. I look up. His mother stands off to the side with a shopping cart and a couple more kids hanging off of it. She is giving me evil eyes. She is Angelina Jolie.

"Sorry, excuse me," I say. I grab my box off the shelf and shuffle away. Wow, I just almost ran over Maddox or Pax—not sure, one of the Southeast Asian ones. I bet people don't normally come so close to her and her brood. *Most people aren't normally tranquilized on a Tuesday afternoon doing laps at Ralphs.* More importantly, what is Angelina Jolie doing at Ralphs? For that matter, what is she doing grocery shopping at all? Huh, I guess she likes to get down with the people's market. Good for her. She looks fragile in person—shorter than I imagined. Much less intimidating than the man-stealing vixen she's always portrayed as, just a mom in a trench coat and some loafers wrangling screaming brats. *That was very normalizing, so whatever,* I think, as I turn the corner. I then see a crowd of people peeking down the aisle and pointing like they've seen a three-headed llama—i.e., less normal. They're on to her in here. At the checkout, it's the same frenzy. Another cashier comes and whispers in the ear of the lady ringing up my three items for sixty bucks.

"Where?" she says and stands on tippy toes.

"Aisle six," the other hisses.

Right by the goddamned rice milk, I think, as she hands me my bags and I go on my oblivious way.

Robbie and I travel to my parents' house in Calgary for Christmas. My dad picks us up at the airport and chauffeurs us back home. It's minus-30 degrees Celsius. We park out front and roll our suitcases inside. I never lived in this house. They bought it a few years after I went off to university. It's their retirement dream home—an attractive duplex along the Bow River. No kids' rooms. A hot tub out back. One guest room in the basement next to my dad's extensive model-train room. My dad is proudly giving Robbie a tour of his latest electrical work lighting up miniature lampposts. I settle us into the April-fresh, cream-colored décor. I hang up my two dresses and Robbie's dress shirts, shove socks and underwear in a top dresser drawer. I'm now fully recovered from my pre-Christmas strep throat, but it will be nice to be taken care of for a minute. Robbie was working most of the time I was sick, unable to ladle soup. Too busy filming porn stars enduring pre-scene enemas, whatnot. A lot of what porn stars go through is distinctly unsexy—the whole constant-maintenance-of-bodily-orifices part. Plucking of ingrown pubic hairs. Bleaching of assholes. Robbie recently told me that one porn star said her pet peeve was discovering toilet paper in another girl's folds while going down on her. I cringe as I place my neatly folded jeans in another drawer. Why am I thinking about this? It's Christmas, for Christ's sake! I shove our suitcases in the laundry room, sprint upstairs like a ten-year-old, and flop down on the couch with my book.

"Want a cup of India Spice, Em?" my mom says.

"Yes, please!" I reply. I plan to take full advantage of my mom doting on me with tea, gluten-free cookies, yoga classes, a trip to the herbalist, and maybe the psychic, who knows. The mom treatment never gets old.

We all sit down for dinner on the first night. Brother Tim is over. He's put on some Lionel Richie. The fire is going. The living room and dining room are on the top floor, which looks out over the freezing river, rushing with great chunks of ice. Snowy pine trees line the far bank along the railroad tracks. The Christmas tree is lit up. It's a winter wonderland in here. My dad pours red wine while my mom lays down plates of Alberta beef, broccoli, and baked potatoes.

Still, the porn world is never far away; like a shy boy at a school dance, it hovers awkwardly behind these types of conversations.

We tick off: "So, are you guys missing winter? How are both sets of parents, Rob? Siblings? How are the wedding plans coming? How is the job search, Em?" Before we arrive at: "And how's work going for you, Rob?"

"It's good, thanks. Getting a little repetitive at this point," Robbie says. Our steak knives audibly glide along the gold-embossed dinnerware.

"Well, I guess you'll be looking forward to the next thing," my dad says matter-of-factly, sipping his Cabernet. "Claire, will you pass the Branston Pickle?"

"Do you want to go cross-country skiing tomorrow?" Tim interjects.

"Yes!" I say. "But I don't think I have skis anymore."

"We can rent them from the outdoor center at the university, then take them to Kananaskis," he says.

"Cool."

The mood livens again with that icky bit of business out of the way. We make ski plans, yoga plans, shopping plans, and dinner plans. For a whole blessed Christ's birthday week, we never revisit the topic again.

Back in LA, Kate pulls up in an electric blue Mustang convertible. She's come for a visit to escape Canadian winter.

"We'll be driving exclusively with the top down," she says, as she bangs through the door with a giant suitcase. "I'm trying to embarrass you as much as possible."

I'm relieved to see Kate. I've been stuck in my head these last months and looking forward to four days of running conversation. We commence immediately by making mango-vodka smoothies, donning sunhats and short shorts, and plopping ourselves on the grass. Our lawn isn't really ideal for sunbathing, given that it is bordered from the sidewalk by only a metal fence. But we don't give a shit. We stretch out on blankets and bear our midriffs to the neighbors because we are northern people and that is the only way we know how to consume sun—like it's the last time we'll ever see it. An old Armenian man in a velour tracksuit looks at us dubiously as he passes with his Chihuahua. It is, after all, January. If you ask me, his choices are equally questionable.

Kate flings off her flip-flops and says, "So, where's Rob?"

"Probably filming some bukkake scene."

"Come again?"

"Haha," I say.

"'Haha' what?

"Oh, I thought you were punning. *Bukkake* is when a bunch of guys stand around jerking off and then ejaculate on someone, usually all over their face."

"Ah, I get it. That's nice. Wow, you really just rattle this shit off now."

"I use the Urban Dictionary a lot. I think it's supposed to be about humiliation. Remember in high school when just spitting or swallowing was a big deal? You couldn't win either way—if you spit you were a prude, swallowed and you were a slut. I wonder if bukkake is all the rage with the teens these days. They've really upped the ante."

"Yikes, I hope not!" Kate says. "One guy ejaculating on me is my limit, and tits only, nobody likes that shit in the eye."

"I hear you. Allowing one guy, let alone ten, to jizz on my eyebrows has never been part of the program."

"Well I'm not into humiliation—remember the 'Do you like that?' guy?"

I know exactly whom she's referring to. A dude she had a huge crush on until they had drunk sex one night in a closet and the whole time he repeated: "Can you feel that? Do you like that?" in a throaty voice. Kate felt like she was starring in his favorite porn, but not in a hot and sexy way. That was the end of that romance.

"Yes, that was unfortunate," I say. Kate shudders. "Maybe it's better if you're prepared, like, before you go to work you look in the mirror and repeat ten times, 'I'm good enough, and gosh darn, people like me!' And then you go get heaps of jizz on your face."

"You couldn't pay me enough. Maybe 10 million," Kate says.

"Maybe they're genuinely into it?" I say.

Kate raises her eyebrows and then shrugs.

"So how are the horses?" I ask, changing the topic. Her eyes light up and she launches into her recent updates. I fill her in on my job search. We chat until the sun ducks behind a building and the temperature drops. By eight o'clock, we are tipsy and exhausted. We talk about going out on the town, but decide that we are too uncool, lazy, old. Instead, we make frozen pizza and curl up on the couch for a movie night.

Kate and I spend three blissful days driving around LA in our lame car. We go to Malibu. Hike Griffith Park to the observatory. We catch a movie and have dinner at The Grove and watch the ridiculous fountain dance to Michael Jackson. Robbie's been busy working, probably more bukkake scenes. He and Matt come and go. We exchange hellos, but frankly, we're too busy to pay much attention to them. Later, boys. This is girls' club time. On her last night, we go for drinks at the Chateau Marmont.

We sit out on the terrace, surrounded by lush greenery in the warm, candlelit darkness. It's a perfect LA night, just cool enough to drape a scarf over your shoulders and call it seasonal fashion. It's a midsummer night's dream out here, even though it's midwinter. A cute waiter darts between tables, forcibly ignoring us. The terrace is half full of tables of two or three. I wonder how many people here are like us—out-of-towners seeking the LA experience. Scant service notwithstanding, this place is glorious. And expensive. We eventually order overpriced vodka sodas and appetizers.

"So how are things with you and Robbie?" Kate asks when our drinks and food arrive.

"Not bad," I say. "It's been a weird time. We're hanging in there."

"You know you can talk to me about whatever, right?"

"Of course. Why?"

"I don't know. I feel like you've been pretty controlled when I ask about how things are out here. Sure you're not creating a high-pressure system in there?" she says, twirling her pointer finger at my head.

I sip my vodka and savor a piece of ahi tuna. I know my friend is on to something, but I'm afraid of revisiting last summer. What is she really asking? Have I assuaged any fears that I'm not marrying a cheater? Or am I cool with my new role as the porn wife here in LA? "I think things are okay," I say.

"That's really convincing. What's bugging you, luv?"

I feel my throat closing up and my eyes watering. Nobody has asked me that recently. Robbie steers clear of talking to me about the job. I think he assumes I'm resolved to it all at this point. But the truth is, I still don't fully understand my myriad feelings. I'm not exactly letting anyone in to help. She grabs my hand across the table.

"Do you think it looks to them like you're breaking up with me?" I say, nodding at the table next to us.

"Yes," she says. "Now tell me what the hell you're thinking."

"Nothing is like I thought it would be, I guess. I'm lonely here. I only have one friend because the other friend I tried to make hit on me. Robbie is gone all day and night filming porn. And I don't even know why that bothers me. I feel like it shouldn't after all this time. But it still does."

"It's okay that it bothers you."

"Is it though, really? I mean, it's his job and who really cares if he films a million cum shots at this point?!" The people at the table next to us glance in my direction. I smile sweetly.

"It won't be forever. How much longer is there to go?"

"Five more years, it feels like. But actually, it might be another four months. They keep bumping back the schedule because of plotlines."

"Four months? It's already been going on for the better part of a year. Wow, that's still a while."

"I know. I never imagined that being engaged would be like this. I'm supposed to feel so certain about things, and instead I feel more jealous and insecure than I did over long distance."

"It's a huge adjustment just moving here, and it really doesn't help that he's filming porn stars all day," Kate says.

"I feel like I always have to hide the fact that it brings up mixed feelings for me because I assume most people would be fine with this."

"Are you kidding me?"

"No."

"Listen, I can tolerate a boyfriend who watches porn from time to time, but I don't want to think about it *every* day. And for the record, many women are not okay with porn, or at least wouldn't be okay with their fiancé filming it. I think probably just pretending that you're cool with all this must be taking up a huge amount of energy."

"I'm exhausted!" I nod. I put my fork down on the plate and slump in my chair. "I guess it was just easier to have porn be compartmentalized and not spill over into other elements of my life."

"I think most people feel that way. Separation of church and state."

"Why do we have these two worlds? The 'woo you and take you on a date' world and then the 'go home and watch some hard-core teenage sluts' part?"

"I don't know." She shakes her head sympathetically. "But we compartmentalize so that everyone doesn't go around living out their baser instincts. So that we can uphold society and marriage and monogamy and maintain a puritanical front."

"Yes, that's all true. So basically we're all fooling ourselves. We're all Dr. Jekyll and Mr. Hyde. Why can't we just be free-loving?"

"What, you want to live on a commune now? Give me a fucking break. Total sexual freedom doesn't really exist without all kinds of messiness." She shudders.

"Ugh, I just don't want to be this high-maintenance," I say.

"Good luck with that."

"Are you making fun of me?" I say, laughing. It feels good to finally express all these feelings. To not swallow back my deep qualms about porn and Robbie's role in it in the name of being an amenable, deferential fiancée. Damn, it's like emotional bukkake. The shit's really coming out now, and it feels great.

"Yes! You *are* high-maintenance. But I love you, and Robbie does too.

"I am? Really?"

She raises her eyebrows at me. "I think you are less high maintenance when you don't feel threatened."

"And why, again, do I feel threatened?"

"Because the porn world is pretty intimidating, Em! There are a lot of really big dildos flying around! It's not something everybody has contact with or even talks about. Our fantasy lives are usually extremely private."

"Right. And this is more, 'Hi, honey. How was the gang bang?' day after day, after day, after day, after day . . ."

"Yes."

"It feels really intense. I feel so compared to these cum-in-the-face-every-five-second girls! And so I silently judge them, feel bad for them, or try to keep up! When did I get so masochistic?"

"Again, do I have to replay your whole life for you? You always pick at the wound. This is intense for you. That's okay. But you probably need to be more honest with yourself and Robbie."

"I thought I had been." I sigh and slug the rest of my drink in one shot.

"By telling him to go ahead and work in a world that you have personal and moral dilemmas with every day?"

"Yes. What else can I do?"

She looks at me deadpan and motions to the sprinting waiter that we'll have another round. He nods.

"You mean ask him to quit?" I say.

"Is it really the end of the world? Wouldn't it solve a few problems, and you two lovebirds could get on with planning happily ever after?"

"And pretend this didn't happen?"

"I'm just saying that you could do yourself an emotional favor and think about the seedier parts of life a little less and your upcoming nuptials a little more. There's nothing inherently wrong with, say, a little time spent mulling over flower arrangements. I'm not telling you to go all Bridezilla, but the wedding is eight months away. Have you even thought about bridesmaids' dresses or cake or seating arrangements?"

"No, I only think about double penetration."

"Right. See, I think maybe there's a happy medium somewhere. Hey, I hate to interrupt this, but I think I see someone I know over there."

"Ryan Gosling?"

"Sadly, no. Just this girl I know from the Florida riding circuit."

The waiter deposits two more cocktails in front of us. "Can we take our drinks over there?" she asks him. He motions to go ahead. "Want to take a breather and go say hi?" she asks me.

"Yes, absolutely."

We make our way around the terrace.

"Leslie?" Kate says, as we get up close, and they erupt into squeals and hellos. Leslie is with a girlfriend as well, a pretty blonde girl who introduces herself as Rachel.

"We were just deep into a talk," Leslie sighs. "I'm trying to convince Rachel to ditch the douchebag she's been sleeping with."

"I know I should," Rachel says and nods somberly.

"He's not going to suddenly want something serious now that he's tasted the goods," Leslie says.

"I work with him," Rachel divulges, looking down into her drink. "We've been sleeping together for a few months, but he never wants to do anything other than hook up late at night."

"Sounds like trouble," Kate says.

"Right?" Leslie says.

"I guess if you want a relationship, then yeah, it sounds like he's not in it for that," I concur.

Rachel nods. "I didn't think I wanted any commitment at first . . ." she says. "Ugh, but now I'm attached. How do I make the switch from just casual?"

"I really don't think you can," Leslie says emphatically.

I space out on my vodka buzz and look around at the other chattering, imbibing patrons. People hover with drinks around tables. It's getting a little louder, drunker, out here. Our increasingly animated conversation is unbearably typical: Girl sleeps with guy and gets attached to him. Guy won't commit. It's the kind of babble that used to make my eyes roll back in my head irretrievably. Except right now I find myself envying the solvability of Rachel's issues. This is the kind of conundrum that a couple of drunk girlfriends can put their heads together on and come up with a solution—ditch the douchebag who won't go out in public with you, voilá! And if Rachel doesn't get it the first time around, a cursory Google search will uncover at least a million advice columns on the subject. Or she can zip over to Barnes and Noble where books on this matter crowd the shelves of the self-help section—*How to Land a Man and Marry Him! How to Make Him Commit! He's Just Not That Fucking into You!*

I have a different conundrum. My man is devoted. He's down to be seen in public with me every dang day of the week. He's into me (at least when he's not doubled over with exhaustion and leg cramps from shooting porn). We plan to marry, spawn kids, maybe build a home in the country and raise some chickens, dogs, whatnot. I have the ring I never thought I wanted. It's right here sparkling in the evening light—a ruby! Shimmering while I clench my cocktail. What self-help genre does my problem fall under? How to marry a man filming porn and not feel like a tight-ass, sexually inadequate, judgmental psycho-bitch and drown my emotions in fermented potatoes? Maybe it simply falls under, How to not care about shit that bothers you. Or, How to look on the bright side and fucking relax. I appreciate what Kate said. But I don't know whether putting my foot down at this late hour serves any point or will just create an even bigger fracture between us. I still think that with the right amount of mental willpower, I can solve this on my own. I chomp an ice cube from the bottom of my now-empty vodka and soda and wince. My teeth hurt from whitening them recently—another bright idea I had in the name of looking hot for my entry into matrimonial bliss. *Clearly I'm focusing on what matters.* Forget about my relationship with the groom, my crooked pearly whites are blinding!

After cocktail number four or six, not sure, the candlelit tables in the distance are a blur and Rachel is texting the douchebag to hook up. We give up. Brad Pitt could plop down on my lap and I'm not too sure I'd recognize him. Kate and I bum a cigarette and the nicotine takes me from buzzed to blotto. We decide to go. It's midnight. Kate's flight is at 10:00 AM tomorrow. I whip my pashmina over my shoulder dramatically, trying to appear pulled together, continental, and accidentally swipe the waiter collecting our credit card slips. He shoots me a bitchy look. I grab the backs of chairs as I stumble along the cobblestones in my heels. How many celebs have bailed on these fuckers? *Here's looking at you, Lindsay.* I guess they have an entourage to hold them up, whereas I just have Kate, who is equally uncoordinated. Goddamned heels. Motherfucking LA winter fashion. I'm much more coordinated in mukluks and a snowsuit.

We leave the Marmont and trudge along on Sunset Boulevard, instantly downgraded from princesses to whores. We hail a cab and make a drive-through pit stop for French fries at Jack in the Box, which I promptly spill all over the car's floor mat. The last thing I remember is Kate smashing me in the arm as I reach down to grab one.

I wake up in bed the next morning registering a sore shoulder and bright midmorning sunshine filtering through the blinds.

"Did Kate make her flight?" I mumble to Robbie, who faces me, sleepy-eyed on his pillow.

"Yeah, I heard her leave a while ago," he says. I reach for the water glass on my bedside table and chug a few mouthfuls. "So do you want to hear crazy?" he continues.

"Sure, what?" I say. My head hurts. I'm parched.

"Do you remember that gonzo scene with Nine where that Montreal girl, Valaria, joined in without permission?"

"Yeah, how could I forget."

"Well, it turns out she gave all three of the other performers gonorrhea."

"Wow."

"I know. Unfortunate."

"*Unfortunate?* That's the understatement of the year for her." I sit up abruptly, ready to hold court. Immediately I realize being upright is too ambitious. I steady myself with one arm. "This is reason number one the porn world comes off as sketchy. What's the rule for testing again?"

"Well she hadn't been tested, remember? But they get tested every twenty-two days. Still, anything can happen in their private lives, or at work, like this scenario."

I rub my hands over my face, forgetting that I'm still wearing makeup until my fingertips meet my crunchy eyelashes. I catch my reflection in the mirror—raccoon eyes, electrocuted hair, inexplicably sporting an angora sweater I was not wearing last night, and nothing else. "How the fuck are condoms not the norm in porn!" I yell, throwing my hands up. "Would people seriously stop watching it just because condoms are not sexy? It's so dumb!"

"Actually, I heard another perspective from a female performer," Robbie says, lying at leisure with one arm propped behind his head. "She said that using condoms for the kind of rigorous penetration they do creates sores that can spread STDs even easier. There's a lot of friction."

"Seriously? What the fuck is lube for?" I say, swinging my legs over the side of the bed and thinking very hard about how I'll get to the shower.

"Anal sex?"

"Haha. Get some condoms and some lube and make the idiot customerbase deal with it. There, done, I just solved the STD crisis. Who are these retards?"

"I think you just called me an idiot and porn producers retards. You're in a really great mood this morning, lovey."

"Well, come on, it's so simple, no?" I pull off my sweater and slowly stand up, testing my proficiency with gravity. It's not great. I have blisters from my misadventures in heels.

Robbie shrugs. "Why don't you get back in bed, sexy? I don't work until tonight. One of our porn stars is hosting some night at a club."

"That's nice!" I say, looking down at him. "You go clubbing with your gonorrhea friends. I'll stay here and try not to saw my feet off or overdose on Tylenol Cold."

"What's going on?"

"Nothing, really," I say, holding the doorframe for support as I pass through it. "Don't worry about me!" I call out from the bathroom as I crank the squeaky hot-water tap. "I just need a shower, some coffee, a lobotomy, and I'll be raring to go."

CHAPTER 11

STAND-INS

Midmorning on a Saturday in February, Robbie and I stand in line at the Alcove Café. We hover in front of a display case that flaunts carrot cakes, fig bars, and double-decker fudge brownies. Maybe later. I stare at the extensive menu. I need salt, sustenance—eggs it is. We shuffle forward, two by two, behind folks in oversized sunglasses jangling car keys and wallets, jonesing for caffeine. We place our order with the frazzled girl at the cash register. I would be frazzled, too, if I had ten people hovering around me at all times. With a feeble smile, she hands us our drinks and a number to take to our table.

The patio is set back from the road and bordered by a low brick wall; a large tree grows within its confines, making the area feel secluded even though it's steps from traffic. We find a spot for two, half shaded by an umbrella. Robbie takes the shade; I sit in the sunny spot and flip down my glasses from my head where they've been acting as a headband. I sip my enormous Arnold Palmer and take in the scene—people wearing wool hats and scarves with their tank tops. Only in LA. I do a scan for celebs. Last time I was here, I saw Kiefer Sutherland, which is officially the least exciting celebrity sighting ever because (a) most of my friends have also spotted him shitfaced on a sidewalk back in Canada at some point or another, and (b) he plays in Robbie's LA hockey league. These factors bring his "wow" factor way down to "whatever." Sorry, Kief.

For the last couple of days, Robbie's been filming at The Exxxotica Expo, which is billed as the "largest event in the USA dedicated to love and sex." This expo, I've gathered, is like any other car or electronics convention, just with more strap-ons and naked chicks. I thought about tagging along one day, since it's a public place and all. Then I reflected on how awesome it would make me feel to see his coworkers in G-strings selling nipple clamps, and reconsidered. I'm tenuously feeling better about life. I've been to my second interview for a job as a personal assistant to an actor, and it looks like I have the position! Yup, I've finally found someone sympathetic enough to sponsor a polite Canadian with two arts degrees. He wants someone to fulfill the vague task of "making his life better." Indeed, it sounded potentially suspect. But after a breakfast interview at the Hollywood 101 Diner, I think he's merely interested in me color-coding his filing cabinet. Fingers crossed.

"I have my first trial day at the new job next week!" I say to Robbie.

"That's so good, my love," he says. "Congrats." We clink beverages. My spinach omelet and Robbie's Benedict arrive. I salt and pepper my eggs, mound of potatoes, and salad. We tuck in. I watch cars pass on Hillhurst Avenue. Our cutlery clinks. I catch a word or two of other people's conversations. As is often the case these days, the silence between us that I used to find refreshing feels loaded.

"So? What's new with you?" I say, not referring to the job in particular, but Robbie goes there.

"Well, Johnny is having a moral dilemma," Robbie says and continues to explain as he cuts into a yolk, flooding it with hollandaise sauce. Johnny Gun is a porn star turned director. His girlfriend, another performer, is pregnant and suddenly not as keen on things like fisting. She wants out of the biz. To boot, she doesn't seem to love having her baby daddy continue to sleep with her former porn-star coworkers. *How odd.* I guess being pregnant is making her see things differently. And want different things. I nod vigorously as he tells me the story.

"Sounds familiar," I say.

"What?" he says, raising his eyebrows dubiously behind his aviator-style Ray-Bans.

"I mean, minus the baby-daddy sleeping with my porn-star friends part! I just mean that planning a future with someone makes you see things differently."

"Remember when you told me you didn't want to get married?" he asks, laughing. I nod. Of course I remember; it was five minutes ago. When Robbie proposed to me eight months ago, it went like this: We were sitting at a crappy tourist restaurant on the main strip in Santa Barbara. The sun was setting. The food was shit. We were thoroughly enjoying each other's company. The booze was flowing and I was going on about my master's thesis, which was a two-hundred-page diatribe about why my generation—children of the Baby Boomers—is so much slower to pass the traditional milestones of adulthood, like getting married, having kids, being gainfully employed, whatnot. More specifically, I was sipping a martini and gesticulating wildly when I said: "I don't know if I ever want to get married! I don't want a lifelong sentence of doing someone's laundry! I'm not that into toddlers!!"

Twenty minutes later, Robbie proposed. He said: "I want to spend my life with you. I'll happily stay home and raise the kids. We'll make up the rules as we go."

I said absolutely, "*Yes, yes, yes.*"

After dinner, we tried to go find a hotel and consummate the thing. But because it was graduation weekend at UC Santa Barbara, everything was booked. We hopped in the Hyundai, hoping to find somewhere along the road—no vacancy. We drove all night, taking an ill-advised detour along Malibu Canyon's high, hairpin turns in the dark. *Oopsie, never trust me with a map.* We pulled up at Russell Avenue at four in the morning excited and delirious and very much in love.

I don't know how it feels to suddenly want out of the porn world while your boyfriend still works in it. But I know something about revising your life plans to make room for someone else. Meeting Robbie, falling for him, and becoming engaged has me considering ideas I was once skeptical of—like everlasting promises. How many times in my twenties did I sip wine with girlfriends and talk about how marriage was a suspect notion? Who wanted to be tied down to one man? We'd all read Erica Jong in Feminist Literature 101, followed by *The Ethical Slut.* We weren't dopes. We knew that any sane woman was daft to entwine happily ever after with a man—to expect him to satiate her mentally and emotionally while also fulfilling her sexually.

Yet here I am, wanting more from Robbie than I ever imagined. I've spent the better part of the last year quite literally waiting around for him, trying to get in his head, to feel secure in his commitment to me with this other world of licentiousness swirling around us. It's not lost on me that porn exists as a means to exercise your sexual fantasies and leave long-term monogamy intact—the very thing we're optimistically signing on to. But why do we need one to prop up the other? Maybe our society only craves hard-core smut because aspiring to monogamy is so ass-backward and fucked up. Maybe it's marriage I should be wary of, and porn is just bringing its inadequacies to the surface. Perhaps we aren't meant to be strapped down to one partner and we should stop forcing the issue once and for all. What's that oft-recited stat again—it doesn't work out nearly half of the time? I can't go a day in this world without reading about the latest cheating scandal—even when I steer way clear of *US Weekly*.

"Em?" Robbie says. Oh right, Robbie, omelets, conversation. "Where did you go?"

"Here! Sorry! So what's Johnny going to do?"

"I'm not sure. I guess they'll find a compromise."

"Right." Compromise. That sounds sensible. Maybe she's okay with him just directing, not performing. Or maybe for her it's about the kind of scenes he does. Who knows? They'll have to determine their own comfort zones. A couple that works in porn probably talks about their sexual boundaries more than most. As I know well, it's easier not to talk about things that make us uncomfortable unless they smack you in the cheekbone. I've been thinking about Kate's idea ever since she left—the whole cut-and-run strategy. I keep *almost* bringing it up with Robbie. Something stops me. What am I really running from if I ask him to quit? Would it solve something or just be a Barbie Band-aid cover-up?

"Any word on how much longer you guys will be filming?" I say, attempting to ascertain how much more of this I'm in for. *Maybe I can just wait it out . . .*

"Michel is trying to resolve all of these dangling plotlines. A few more months at least," he says.

"So you could, hypothetically, still be shooting porn by our wedding in August?" I say, half joking. "Move over, Aunt Trudi, make way for Madison X."

"Doubtful," he says earnestly. He swallows his last bite and pushes his plate aside, reclining with a manly grunt and tummy rub. I nod.

"Want to talk about our honeymoon?" I say. We're thinking road trip in France. A few days in Paris, Provence, and then maybe some time along the Mediterranean. Planning our itinerary is my job, since he's otherwise occupied. I pull up a few i-escape listings on my phone.

"Okay, there's an amazing-looking *auberge* in Saint-Rémy," I say. "Check this out." I show him a picture of a courtyard with a fountain. He smiles and slides his chair around the table. He puts his hand on my knee. Yup—this is much, much easier to talk about.

The next day I am napping after a rigorous yoga class when Robbie comes home. I wake to find him sitting at the end of the bed looking at me.

"Hi," I say.

"Hi, sweetheart."

"How's it going?"

Robbie bends over and takes off his shoes, then slides onto the bed next to me.

"Good," he says. "It looks like I'm going to be going on a trip for the show. Madison X and her husband, Dan, are travelling to the Dominican Republic to film some porn."

"Oh." Madison is the lesbian fetish star whose husband films and directs her. I can picture her instantly—some studded dog collar around her neck, sparkly eye shadow, the weird *Girls Next Door* mix of baby-pink innocence and hard-core behavior. "I guess that's nice for you," I say.

"Yeah." He lies back on the pillow next to me. "I leave next Tuesday and will be gone for a week. I wish you could come."

"Me too." I turn toward him on the pillow. "That's over Valentine's Day."

"It is? Oh crap, I didn't even think of that. Good thing you don't care about Valentine's Day." He glances at me with a smirk on his face. Truthfully, I have never gone in for long stems and truffles. But on our first V Day together as a couple, Robbie made it his mission to prove me wrong. He picked me up from the sushi restaurant where I was bartending at the time and whisked me to his apartment. Then he drew me a bath filled with red rose petals, served me warm brownies with raspberries and cream, and doted on me with a back massage while I sipped red wine. I'd be lying if I said I didn't enjoy the experience. Of course, now he's raised the bar, only to follow it up with shooting other people filming porn during a tropical getaway without me. Times have changed.

"Yeah, good thing," I say. "Why the Dominican, not Malibu?"

"I guess we're supposed to scout local talent at San Juan strip clubs for Madison to film with."

"Seriously?"

"Yeah."

"They're just going to walk into strip clubs and say, 'Hi, want to come film some porn with us?' What about the whole STD-testing thing? What about there being a difference between what a stripper does and what a porn star does—how are they handling all of that?"

"I don't know. I didn't ask."

"You didn't think of any of that? Isn't it kind of a stretch to just offer strippers some cash to make the leap to porn? What the fuck? Who are these assholes?"

Robbie sighs. "Sorry, no, none of that occurred to me. I was just thinking about the trip."

"Well, lucky you! Sorry to annoy you with my overthinking or, for that matter, just considering any of these factors at all."

"Hey, what's that supposed to mean? I'm the insensitive jerk? This is my job, Emily. I'm not an investigative reporter. Besides, maybe these strippers want to shoot porn. I don't know. But I'll find out next week, won't I? Why are you jumping down my throat? I am so sick of this bullshit from you."

"It's bullshit for me to take issue with this? Okay, if you say so." I get up off the bed and grab a hoodie from the closet.

"Where are you going?"

"Away from here! From this shit. Have fun in the motherfucking Dominican," I say and grab my purse as I walk through the living room and out of the apartment. The screen door clacks pathetically behind me. I could use the heft of broad oak. I slap down Russell Avenue in my flip-flops, turn left on Western, and right again on Hollywood Boulevard. I don't know where I'm going. But I know that this has to be one of the ugliest neighborhoods in America. I pass a boarded-up nightclub, an adult-video store, a halfway house, and a run-down corner store advertising lottery tickets. An empty Jamba Juice container tumbles down the sidewalk next to me. Bits of broken glass fill the cracks in the street. I take a seat at a bus stop and wipe the tears from behind my sunglasses. I dial Hilary on my phone and decide to keep walking west because I'm getting looks from strangers.

"I just had a huge fight with Robbie," I say.

"Oh no! How come? I'm just leaving work. Do you want to meet up?"

"Yes, please. It was about his job. Again. I'm so tired of this, Hil," I mumble. Tears continue to cascade down my cheeks.

"Where are you?"

"Walking west on Hollywood."

"Turn around and walk toward my apartment. I'll come meet you. Everything will be okay."

We hang up and I do as I'm told, retracing my steps and then walking through Thai Town. I pass more ugly strip malls, decrepit liquor stores, tacky nail salons. I don't want to live here in this hideous neighborhood. I don't want to make up with Robbie and kiss him goodbye as he goes on his porn trip. I don't want to be a goddamned Hollywood personal assistant. I don't want any more sunny days, gridlock traffic, celebrity sightings. Fuck LA. I've had it and I want to go home. I don't even know if I want to be a wife anymore. I'm not sure I'm cut out for the supporting role after all, or if I even believe that anyone can make it together forever. Who are we to think our love is stronger than this epically flawed system? What kind of start to a marriage is this?

"I give up," I say to Hilary as I open the car door and slouch into the Mini.

"Me too," she says. "Work was brutal. Where to—Arizona? New Mexico?" Her sentiment makes me smile. Instead we stop off for a bottle of Jack Daniel's and a pack of American Spirits and climb the stairs to her apartment. We sit at her counter, pour two glasses on ice, and proceed to chain-smoke. I give her the rundown on the Dominican trip, and she agrees that it's sketchy.

"Why don't they just film something with porn stars in the system here?" she says. It's not like they couldn't pretend to be in the Dominican with strippers. Throw up some extra palm trees and hammocks or some shit."

"I don't know. I guess 'reality porn' is all the rage now, just like *The Real Housewives* of wherever-the-fuck."

"Yeah, but it does seem unnecessarily risky and exploitative. Is he going to put his foot down?"

"It sure doesn't sound like it. It feels like another wedge between us when we really don't need one, you know?" I exhale smoke across her small kitchen where we are sitting on barstools. The nicotine is giving me a headache and making me feel nauseated, but I don't care. The pain is comforting. "So much for the detoxifying benefits of yoga," I joke. Hil laughs.

"It doesn't really sound like Robbie, not to see any of this from your perspective," she says.

"I don't know what sounds like Robbie anymore."

"Really?"

I shrug. "We seem to be coming from really different places."

"I think you guys just need a break from all this." She goes to the fridge to dig out some sustenance to accompany our substances. She finds bread, cheese, mayonnaise, tomatoes, and hot sauce. "You know," she says, loading two slices in the toaster, "it is a bit like guns in my relationship."

"Guns?"

"Yeah, Tucker is really into hunting. He even owns a gun, and as you know, I couldn't disagree more with having firearms in the house. I do not believe in the 'right to bear arms.' But he *actually* does. It's so middle American, so weird."

"Is that going to be a problem?"

"I'm not sure," she says, clearly considering it while buttering toast. "It's a pretty fundamental difference. It might be. I guess I'll find out."

We eat our perfunctory meal, drink more, smoke more. I text Robbie to say I'm safe at Hilary's, talk tomorrow. He doesn't text back.

I wake up at 11:00 AM in all my clothes. Hilary has gone to work. I haven't slept this late in ages—no, wait, that other hangover was just a few days ago. I splash my face with cold water and make a coffee, call Rob.

We have a brief conversation. He says he'll come pick me up. I look out the window at Sunset Boulevard. The day is grey for once. The Mexican restaurant across the way is already filling up with lunch customers. The thought of a burrito makes me want to barf. Instead, I grab my purse and decide to order take-out sandwiches and sodas from the Italian deli downstairs. As I climb in the car, I hand Robbie one—a prosciutto-and-Parmesan peace offering. We've both had time to cool down. He went out with Matt to a bar last night. We're both bleary-eyed. We sit outside Hilary's apartment. It seems implicit that we can't go anywhere before speaking. Our home feels like a minefield. Robbie unwraps the wax paper on his sandwich and takes a bite.

"This is good," he says.

"I'm glad." I look down at my own bocconcini-basil panini. I don't have an appetite yet. "Where do we go from here?" I say.

"We go on," he says between mouthfuls.

I turn and watch him chew. "I feel like accepting this job means accepting everything about this world, and that's not how I feel. I still want to talk about these things," I say.

"But you don't talk about them," he says. "You say nothing for months and then bite my head off out of nowhere. It's not fair."

"Sometimes I do feel fine about it all. And then something strikes me the wrong way, and I revert to all my old feelings about how fucked-up this all is."

"That's okay, you don't have to feel completely resolved about porn, but you take it out on me. You get so angry, Emily. This hasn't been easy for me either."

I nod and stare down at my Lululemon pants. They are four years old and starting to pill at the seams; they've had a good run. I know I've been a nightmare, which doesn't mean I know how to stop. I don't express myself, for fear of being psycho and unlovable, and then I go and make it worse—amplify it all, manifest my own worst nightmare. I'm scared that once he sees all of these parts of me he'll run for the hills, which is ridiculous because he's here, now, eating a sandwich and trying to talk it out despite yet another hissy fit. I am the one who runs.

"I'm sorry I stormed out," I say.

"Thank you. What's with that?"

"I don't know. I guess I have a pretty strong flight reflex. I'm afraid of what will happen if I stay. I might say things I can't take back."

"Are you always going to cut and run?"

"I don't know."

"Do I have to keep you tethered to the house with ten kids?"

"You know I'd just buy a school bus and hit the road."

"Yeah, I know." We are silent for a minute.

"I don't feel like we see eye to eye these days," I say.

"I guess maybe we don't," he says. "None of this is as big a deal for me as it is for you."

His comment hurts. I try to take it for what it is. It's easy to want people to be upset *with you*. So many arguments are just about the stubborn desire for someone to accept your point of view as their own. We battle it out over semantics, when really we just want to be heard. Conceding the point is actually secondary. It's harder to consider that we just might not see eye to eye, ever. To accept it and move on. Is that okay in this context—to agree to disagree? Am I okay with him participating in something I morally oppose? My head hurts too much to answer that right now.

"Should we go home?" he says, putting a hand on my knee. I nod. He starts the car, pulls a U-turn on Sunset, and we drive back to our apartment. Today, I don't have the answers. For now, all we can agree on is taking the day off.

A couple of days later, Robbie is recounting his afternoon to me. It's work-related, of course. After our porn-inspired shake-up, we've settled back into status quo and I'm feeling generous, cool, above it all. *Shit can't touch me* is the attitude I'm trying to take. I push back the little voice that scoffs at me for falling back into old patterns.

"Then some guy burst into the studio and said, 'Johnny, we need your cock'," Robbie says, delivering it like a punchline. I laugh, not because I find it that funny right now, but because Robbie's enthusiasm indicates that I should. I encourage him, "Ha! No way. Why did they need his 'cock'?"

"Well, Johnny was just supposed to be directing, right? But the camera guy in the studio next door apparently double-punched the cum-shot scene."

"Double-punched?" I say. "Is that another humiliation technique, like a Tahitian face mask?"

"No, what's that?"

"It's when you shit on someone's face, wrap it in Saran-wrap, and then punch them." The look on Robbie's face is worth having actually described this twisted act out loud. I feel mildly superior that I know this and he doesn't.

"No! That's disgusting. Where did you learn that?"

"I've been Googling a lot," I shrug.

Robbie laughs. "Okay, well, this has nothing to do with shitting on anyone's face." He shakes his head, clearly imagining it. "Wow, that's even too nasty for me. No, a double punch is when you hit the record button and then forget that the camera is on, and then hit it again so that you've actually stopped recording. Anyway, they needed a stand-in."

"Wow, any old cock will do, I guess."

"We filmed him jerking off to some porn to get hard for the scene."

"No pressure," I say, helping myself to avocado salad, wondering what that scene would be like. I find it mildly arousing to imagine Robbie filming this guy masturbating to porn to get hard for an actual porn shot. Actually, it sounds like the setup for a plotline in a gay film. I make a mental note to tell Robbie to pitch it to Jet Set Productions.

"Yeah, he was annoyed that we were following him. Once he was hard, we went into the other studio and filmed him cum on the girl's tits and face."

"Charming."

"But there wasn't enough cum, so they added a bit of sunscreen on her cheeks for effect."

"Okay, really? That just seems gratuitous. Do they always do that?"

Robbie shrugs. "Sometimes."

"Why do guys want to see sooo much cum, anyway?" I no longer find the situation mildly arousing. Instead, this cum-on-the-face theme, which seems to be a standard device in the scenes that Robbie films, tests my shit-can't-touch-me façade.

"Why do you say 'guys'?" Robbie asks, his defenses alerted.

"Well, the director was a guy, wasn't he?"

"Yeah."

"And the intended audience is still mostly guys, so . . ."

"I guess it's just kind of, you know—the evidence," he says, sounding unconvinced himself.

We've had this discussion before. I find the face shots demeaning. I don't want to rehash an old argument, but my hackles are starting to come up. The shit *is* touching me. I don't want to end up with the equivalent of a psychological Tahitian face mask, and I don't want to be at odds with him *yet again,* so I back off. Try to recoup my too-cool-for-school attitude by playing a different card.

I smile. "It's so much easier for girls to fake their orgasms. Maybe they should actually get paid less than guys. Their job is kind of easier."

"They don't always fake them," Robbie says, sounding affronted. I raise my eyebrows at him. He chews a mouthful of pesto linguine. "What? They don't," he says. "I'm not saying they're all real . . . but sometimes they are."

"You think you can tell by watching?" He shrugs. "Oh my God! You do, don't you?" I tease. "That's so sweet, honey."

"No, not always," he blurts. "But you can definitely tell when a girl is actually into it. It's way more of a turn-on."

"Oh, I bet you get fooled all the time, mister."

"Okay, I used to think more orgasms were real, before this job. But now I can tell the difference."

"If you say so, sweetheart—you're the psychic orgasm reader. I'll let you have your suspension of disbelief." I take a bite of my food, eye him playfully.

"Don't be a jerk," he says, laughing, and throws a cherry tomato from his plate to mine. "You're the one who needs a whole made-up romance novel to get turned on."

I'm beginning to enjoy myself again, to feel less righteous and indignant. My playful condescension is working. We're having fun instead of fuming. Talking about porn instead of arguing over points of view. *Crisis averted.*

"That's not true, actually," I say. "The times I've watched porn lately, I think I've been more turned on by just seeing body parts than needing to believe in the scene. I already know the fantasy is bullshit. It's usually so poorly executed anyway. And when I fantasize in my head, it's usually just a collection of images; I don't actually play out scenes from *The English Patient*, believe it or not."

"You've watched porn lately?"

"Yeah, a bit. Since there wasn't an office Christmas party, I had to get to know your coworkers somehow."

"True." Robbie smiles at me and I can tell he's happy we're having a nonconfrontational conversation. This is how it can be—just jokes. Just teasing, talking, nobody taking offense. I'm happy with the moment too. I get up from the table and start clearing the dishes. I wonder how preggo girlfriend feels about Johnny being a stand-in. My guess is that it's one of those things you slide under the carpet, since she'll probably never watch that scene and say, "Hey, honey, isn't that your dick? When did you film that?" Or will she? I shake my head at the thought.

"What's up?" Robbie says, following me into the kitchen.

"Nothing," I say. "Want to walk to Baskin-Robbins?"

"Yes. Leave all this. You cooked, I'll clean after." He brings his plate to the kitchen sink, stands next to me, and leans in. We kiss, then leave the apartment and stroll down the street.

We both order the same: mint chocolate chip, except he has his in a cone and I take mine in a cup. Then we stroll back toward home in silence. The setting sun is casting everything in a hazy light, making even the decrepit buildings look kind of pretty.

"I have a really early flight on Monday," he says. "I can probably take a cab so that you don't have to bring me."

"So you're going? To the Dominican?"

"Yeah, you knew that?"

"I guess I thought things were undecided after the other day. Did you get to talk to Michel about what they're going to be filming?"

Robbie sighs. "No, I'm not going to. I don't really think it's any of my business. This week is $3,000 of work, and we need the money. It's not my job to police what they film."

I don't want to argue again, I really don't. "That's not the only way to see things," I say quietly.

"What?"

"I mean *Webdreams* is capitalizing on this sketchy plotline, the same way they did with the Nine and Valaria situation. It makes good TV, which makes good ratings and advertising money, but it's not very ethical."

"What about that show I worked on last year? *True Beauty.* You didn't ask me not to film that." He's talking about a show where so-called beautiful people are put in situations where their inner beauty is put to the test. Inevitably, people trash-talked and backstabbed and generally made fools of each other and themselves.

"I guess that seemed more harmless."

"It's because this is about sex that it bugs you. But it's no different. This is what I do and it pays our bills. It pays for our meals. It paid for that ring you're wearing."

"Hey, that's not nice," I say, looking down at my ruby. "I didn't ask you to film porn and buy me a fancy ring. And you know, you sound like a meth dealer."

"It's not as clear-cut as you're trying to make things right now," he says, not amused. "I don't think you're seeing the big picture. It's really not like you to draw such hard lines about things."

"Well, maybe I'm changing."

We enter the apartment together in silence. Robbie is not only going on this trip, he's making a point of not budging. There's nowhere for me to run. So I sit on the couch while he goes to the kitchen to clean up. I eat the rest of my melting green ice cream with my tiny pink spoon. I stare at the wall and listen to the dishes clank in the kitchen, wondering if our moments of seeing eye to eye will ever last longer than an hour.

The next evening, Robbie tells me we're going somewhere, to get in the car. It's a surprise. We drive through West Hollywood, turn south on La Cienega, and continue for miles. He eventually pulls over into a parking lot. I have no idea where we are. We hop out and walk along the sidewalk and into a bicycle shop full of snazzy low riders.

"Pick out whichever one you want," Robbie says. "Happy Valentine's Day."

"Seriously?"

"Yeah, I know you miss biking."

It's true. Back in Montreal, and during grad school in Vancouver, I biked everywhere on my ten-speed, Lazy Sue. But she was in such rusted-out disrepair that I abandoned her in a friend's basement before moving here, rather than pay to ship her. I've missed her; she held meaning between Robbie and me. The night we first hooked up, he doubled me home—all drunken six-feet-two of him managing to stay upright on teensy Sue for fifteen blocks. I balanced on the seat in a miniskirt, legs extended to either side. We stopped and made out at every intersection. A week after our night together, he wanted to see me again but didn't have my number. Nor did he want to surprise me at my bartending job (which he correctly intuited would have annoyed the shit out of me). So he left a note on Sue parked outside the restaurant. It said:

> ~~I had a really amazing time last week, would really love to see you again. Call me.~~
> Rob 555-9243
> (too desperate)
> ~~I had so much fun last week! Let's do it again!~~
> Rob 555-9243
> (too exuberant)

Hey, girl. You should call me sometime.
Rob 555-9243
(too flippant)
Hey, had a fun time last week. Be good to see you again.
Rob 555-9243

I was sold. Our romance continued. So this gesture is fitting. Sweet. The unsaid understanding is that I will cuddle up with my new bike while he goes to the Dominican over Valentine's Day to shoot porn. *Awww.* I don't know how I feel about being paid off, so to speak, but I don't want to ruin this moment. It is really thoughtful. What I actually wish for Valentine's Day is that he'd stay here, not go film porn.

We browse around the shop. I keep lingering on a yellow one with a banana seat and six gears. The sales guy—a heavily tattooed skater type—asks me if I want to take it for a ride. I do. Out on the sidewalk, he adjusts the seat and mirrors for me. I pull away from Robbie and pedal along in the sunshine. I think about just continuing south, maybe turning west until I hit the ocean. The fat tires bump along like a Cadillac. She isn't my old ten-speed; she's more LA, more of a cruiser. I go two, three, four blocks. I can't actually just disappear as I want to; I turn around in the next intersection and return to the shop.

"I love her," I say, pulling up to Robbie and the sales guy, now helping another customer with a trial run.

"We'll take it," Rob says to the dude. He nods. "What are you going to name her?" Robbie asks me as we make our way to the checkout.

"Well, it's the bike that porn bought," I say. "So, Lazy Sue 2.0: Slutty Sue."

He nods as he hands over his credit card.

"Thank you," I say. I want to say: *This doesn't change everything. I'm still mad, even though I'm kind of happy right now.* I feel like a bratty child who has been bought off with a trip to the candy store. I stuff the words in my mouth and chew.

"You're welcome, my love."

We drive northeast through LA with Slutty Sue strapped into the trunk. We don't say much. I'm resigned to what's happening, if not resolved.

The next day, I wake up to Robbie kissing me goodbye at 4:00 AM. It's still dark out. I hear his suitcase roll across the wood floor. The front door opens and shuts three times as he loads gear into the taxi. The key turns in the lock. A minute later, the car doors close and the cab hums down Russell Avenue. He's gone.

CHAPTER 12

MASOCHISM

The Dominican sun beams high overhead. Humid air caresses Robbie's bare arms and legs. He walks along a cobblestone pathway with Madison X and her husband, Dan; they are scouting a hotel location to shoot porn—in particular, her getting tied up, whipped, dominated, and fist-fucked by two other women. Madison is dressed in skintight short shorts, a crop top, and has a ponytail sticking out of a baseball cap. Palms grow in beds of mulch on either side of the path, separating passersby from poolside vacationers. It's only eleven in the morning, but bikini-topped waitresses brandish frothy beers and colorful cocktails. The servers balance like flamingos in their wedge sandals as they lean down, depositing drinks onto tables with a smile. Robbie heaves a thirty-pound camera onto his right shoulder and pulls focus. He briefly registers the pain in his muscles but knows it will subside, fade into the background along with the awareness of his feet sweltering in work boots, his thirst, his hunger, and the passing time. He steps back, one boot into the mulch, as he zooms in on the hotel manager, who is conversing with Dan.

"We have a 100 percent repeat return rate," he boasts. He's a squat man clad in an oversized Hawaiian shirt and cargo shorts. He turns left at the end of the pathway, leading them toward a cluster of freestanding bungalows. They aren't particularly posh or even ocean-side. In fact, the grounds are modest compared to the palatial hotels they passed on their way here. What distinguishes this collection of tropical abodes from the next is that the room price—close to $2,000 a night—includes the services of a prostitute. Two lithe, sarong-clad girls exit one of the neighboring bungalows; they whisper something to each other and turn away from the camera.

"Please don't film our patrons or staff," the manager says to Rob as he unlocks a hotel room door. Robbie nods. The eclectic gang crowds into the clean, white, open-concept room and looks around—a bed, two plush armchairs around a coffee table by a mini-fridge, and a large whirlpool bathtub. The air-conditioning is brisk, refreshing. A picture of an electric tropical sunset is displayed in a dark wooden frame above the bed.

"This is really great," Dan says. "When would it be possible for us to shoot here?"

"How long will you take?"

"Just an afternoon. Noon to six. In and out." The pun is entirely lost on him.

They settle on next Tuesday. Robbie pans to Madison.

"It's so perfect, honey!" she squeals. She kicks off her platform flip-flops and exuberantly hops onto the bed. She crawls across it, glittery pink toes stuck in the air. She bounces up and down on all fours.

"You can do me like this, Baby!" she says, mimicking the rocking-back-and-forth motion of doggie style. Then she crawls over to the headboard and grabs it with her hands, lifting up onto her knees and looking back at her audience. "And here, while I watch the sunset!" She giggles and cries out: "Oh, baby! Yeah, baby!" as she plants her cheek into the clichéd vista.

Dan nods in wholehearted agreement."Yes, sweetie. It's the perfect place to shoot porn."

I am on my knees in the kitchen trying to clean years' worth of grime off the floor tiles around the stove. It's amazing how I go through most of my days not noticing how completely disgusting it is down here. Then every so often, on a cleaning rampage, I make it my mission. I zone in on the imperfections. I scrub despite the fact that even with bleach and scouring pads, it will never be pristine. This apartment is too old, too scuffed, too many times repainted. I dip my brush into the soapy water and go to town on a line of browned grout. I hate wearing rubber gloves—they insulate my sweaty hands, make me claustrophobic. I'd rather bathe in toxic chemicals; my hands now have a whitish film. It can't be good. Oh well.

I received an email from Sam this morning. It said: "Hey, man. How's things? Coming through town for a show. Want me to put you on the guest list?"

Sam is the only guy I know who refers to me as "man." I find it endearing. I wonder if he does it with all the girls. Sam plays the drums, and I've heard through the grapevine that his band is doing well. They're making a real go of it, which makes me smile. It's fun to watch friends you knew who jammed in crappy apartments make it to big stages. I wrote back: "Things is good. I'd love to come. Where? When?"

He replied in under a minute: "Tomorrow 10:00 PM, Spaceland. I'll put you down plus one. See you there, man."

The thought of seeing Sam still gives me butterflies—just one or two slow flutterers. I guess some things never fully fade. I find the idea comforting at the moment. It distinguishes all the feelings that do pass from the few that abide. We all have maps of heartstrings connecting us to one another, some thick, some thin, forever forming and vanishing. Sam's is now thin, just barely existent. A much broader tie connects me to Robbie in the Dominican. *Hence the cleaning rampage to pass the time.* He's filming at an all-inclusive sex resort this morning and a strip club this afternoon. When he told me their itinerary last night on the phone, I asked him why throwing a brothel into the mix was necessary. He said they want a location where they can film poolside or under some palm trees, and at this type of resort, anything goes. In fact, the patrons would surely enjoy the perk of live porn, on-site, no laptop required!

"Oh," I said. "That actually has its particular logic." All-inclusive sex resorts, strip clubs—what's next on the business trip itinerary, dear? I didn't even bother to ask. I just hung up the phone and stared at the fucker. On to my favorite game: how to distract my brain from playing out every minute detail of Robbie's day. I dump the bucket of grey water down the drain; my hands look eighty-five years old, as weathered and grey as my heart feels. I think I'll ask Hilary if she wants to be my plus one tomorrow, since my other plus one is distinctly MIA.

Robbie enters the strip club in the early evening. The room is dark and takes a minute to adjust to from the waning sunny day outside. A typical strip club reveals itself—a bar, a stage; booths line the wall. It's currently empty of patrons. A group of ten or so girls who've been biding time on barstools swarm the crew as they enter. The strippers offer up coquettish looks and bargain-price lap dances. The crew takes refuge in a U-shaped booth. Robbie sits on the inside. They aren't allowed to film inside the club, let alone buy lap dances, so they order Cokes—hold the ice—and shoot the shit.

Madison and Dan talk to two girls—look-alike sisters with jet-black hair, perky teenage tits, and curvaceous bodies sheathed in spandex. Loud Latin techno music blares. The lights dance with the music on stage, showcasing no one. It's too early. Too dead. One by one, the strippers abandon Robbie and the crew when they realize they are not there to be entertained. Most of the showgirls sidle back to the bar, but a few crowd Madison and Dan to see what they are talking to the sisters about: whether the girls are interested in filming porn next Tuesday. They are.

The sisters don't have IDs on them but swear they can produce them by tomorrow. They arrange to meet at a café and go over the details. Madison skips with excitement as she and the crew all leave, mission accomplished. Robbie heaves the camera up onto his shoulder and films the exterior of the club. The walls are black and shiny. Madison strikes a pose in the reflective surface. She arches her back, sticks her chest and ass out like a trucker mud flap. Robbie holds focus on her as he walks a semicircle, capturing the performance from different angles.

"Watch out, Dominican, Madison X is gonna rock your world!" she yells.

I stand on our bed posing in the dresser mirror. Reflexively, I tilt my head to the right, cock my hip, and make my mirror, kissy-face. I'm in knee-high boots and a short, black, wool dress for the concert tonight. It's the fourth outfit change; I decide I look pretty good. The regular yoga and occasional, embarrassing sweatathons I've been doing on the

Elliptical to Justin Timberlake are paying off. Thanks, JT! With the right amount of resistance to potato products, I may not have to wear Spanx to my wedding after all. Hilary is picking me up in ten. I run through the house collecting my things like a lunatic. The apartment is messy in Robbie's absence. I find it helps to have a witness to be tidy. Left to my own devices, I generally leave a flurry of clothes and belongings in my wake. At least I can eat off the kitchen linoleum! At the moment, I can't find my damn keys anywhere. I try every purse I've used in the last week, my gym bag—nothing. In the meantime, I collect a blazer from the back of the couch, lip gloss from the top of the bookshelf, and pull an old, stale pack of American Spirits from the freezer. I feel I may need to smoke later. On my sprint through the kitchen, I spot my keys tucked under the lip of a dirty plate on the counter. *Well done, Emily.* I take a glug from last night's half-drunk glass of red wine. It tastes like shit.

Hil and I zip through Silver Lake in her Mini. We arrive right on time, which in the world of indie concerts is always much, much too early. We valet the car, point out our names on the guest list, and then hit the bar. Hilary orders a Jack Daniel's on the rocks. I get a pint of beer. We perch at a tall table in a dimly lit area adjacent to the stage.

"Kind of a trip to see Sam's band come through LA," I say.

"For sure. It's so great for them. So great for Sam," she concurs. On cue, I see him walk out of a back room by the entrance and talk to the cute doorgirl. I watch him smile and tip his head back in laughter. He looks good in a button-down shirt and skinnier jeans than I remember. *All the boys are doing it these days, even the ones who really shouldn't.* But he pulls it off nicely. He has a scruff of beard and a ratty ball cap on, no doubt to cover his receding hairline. Robbie, too, has progressively extending power alleys and a bald spot. I guess tall, white, bearded, bald men are my thing—how original. I watch Sam lean one elbow on the counter, probably saying something flirtatious. He's good at that—funny and coy, just the right amount of forward. He disappears back through the door.

"I just saw Sam over there," I say to Hil, who has her back to him.

"Oh yeah," she spins her head around.

"I think he went backstage again," I say.

"Do you want to go say hi?"

"Nah, I'll wait." I take a deep slug of beer. I feel nervous. I don't know why; I'm just here to support an old friend who I happened to date for five years.

The room fills up as the first band plays a few songs. I'm not crazy about them—too much rocking out and not enough melody for my taste. It's now stuffy and cramped inside, so Hilary and I take a break out front. She lights a cigarette. The night is crisp by LA standards. My wool dress is too warm inside, but perfect out here. I cool to a normal temperature before putting my blazer on.

"Everything okay with you?" Hilary asks me.

"Yeah, I'm just hot. Is it insanely muggy in there?"

She shrugs. "You know me, I'm always cold." It's true. Hilary can go to Bikram yoga in a cashmere sweater and not break a sweat. It's not fair. As we stand among a small crowd in the parking lot, one of Sam's bandmates walks by.

"Hey," I say, touching his arm lightly as he passes.

"Oh, hey, Emily," he says, with friendly surprise. "Long time no see. Does Sam know you're here?"

"Yeah!" I say loudly. "I mean, no," I backtrack. "He invited me, but I haven't seen him yet."

"Cool," he says, looking at me sidelong. "Well, I'll tell him you're out here. Good to see you."

"You too!"

"Are you on Adderall?" Hilary asks me.

"Fuck me, no," I sigh. "I don't know what's wrong with me. I feel really nervous, like this is a blind date or something, which it's not at all! Don't judge."

"I wouldn't," she says, and butts out her cig with her pointy-toed suede boots. "We all have skeletons."

Robbie crosses my mind for a second as we walk back inside and into the crowd. He must be knee-deep in a stripper/porn-star lesbian jungle fuckathon by now—whips, studded collars, and massive black dildos everywhere. I've told him not to bother calling tonight. The logic: if we don't speak, there's no way to fight. I need more beer.

The stripper sisters meet Madison and Dan at the designated café, which is more of a roadside cantina. The day is scorching. The four of them sit at a shaded table; Robbie stands off to the side filming from a tripod. The director watches the action on the monitor. The girls direct their attention to Dan, who speaks some Spanish, and explain that they cannot provide their IDs because they left them at home. Home is a town several hours away. He tells the girls that they can't film together unless they show IDs.

"What did they say?" Madison asks, tugging Dan's arm.

"They don't have IDs," Dan reiterates.

"Oh no! But they're so hot!" she says. "I want to do a scene with them. Can they go get it?"

The sisters say they will try their best to have IDs by tomorrow. They'll call then. It doesn't sound promising. The girls leave. Madison pouts. Dan attempts to make her feel better by ordering hamburgers and sodas. Then, ever the businessman, he strategizes what to do next.

Demonstrating a valid ID, or at least the semblance of it, is a rule they won't break. Where else can they find some last-minute porn stars? Should they call a talent agency? Go back to the strip club? Something needs to happen fast. They're booked to shoot at the all-inclusive sex resort tomorrow. They decide to cancel the hotel to take the pressure off, and then scout another location.

Robbie packs up the equipment. They all load into a van and drive to an oceanside vista obscured by a natural bluff. Madison hops out of the rental, bouncy again with the promise of still accomplishing their goal—an orgy in the jungle. Robbie climbs up the bluff to shoot the scene from above.

"It's so perfect, baby!" Madison squeals. "Look! It's made for us. You can string me up here!" She stands between two palm trees a few feet apart and demonstrates a spread-eagle pose. The trunks make perfect, natural restraint holds. Things are looking up.

I am squatting to pee in a grimy bathroom stall with arms extended to either side like a gymnast recovering from a vault landing. I hold the handrail with my left hand and press my right palm against a cold, graffitied wall. Why can I never get the hang of balancing like this? I can do a headstand, but not this maneuver. It takes all my focus to relax enough to pee but not become so relaxed that my ass sags onto the urine-splashed seat. Sam's band is about to come on stage. I'm tipsy and wanted to check my reflection first. Knowing me, I'll have smeared mascara on my cheeks or have left a film of beer head on my upper lip—sexy! I exit the stall, run my hands under the tap, and apply lip gloss in the oxidized mirror. All clear, from what I can make out. I push back through the crowd to where Hilary stands close to the stage. Sam walks on and sees me as he sits at his drum kit. He gives me a wink; I smile back. *Crap, I'd forgotten how sexy he is up there.* When we were breaking up, I had to boycott his shows because every time I saw him in bright lights, I fell back in love with him. I'm starstruck again. They start with a tune I know. Hil and I bop along. During the song break, she excuses herself to go call Tucker. I stand alone in the crowd feeling blissful. I feel like my old self—someone who doesn't constantly feel threatened or afraid of losing everything, a girl who hops up and flies off to Peru and Spain alone, just because! I didn't used to worry so much. I just assumed everything would work out great, or at least okay, because it mostly always had. Where is that me now—the girl who just trusts?

The lead singer says hello to his LA audience and introduces the second song, called "boyfriends and girlfriends." It starts slowly, dreamily, and builds. Then it slows, almost stopping, and builds again. I want it to last. Hilary edges back into the crowd and taps me on the shoulder. She whispers to me that she's leaving; she's tired and wants to see Tucker. I say no problem. I'll take a cab home. I'm actually happy to be left alone. I feel good on my own tonight. Alone, I know where the rest of the world ends and I begin. I'm not obsessing about someone else's reality, for once. I'm just me—here, now, swaying in an anonymous crowd. Even if a little beer buzz and nostalgia are helping this independent feeling along.

The show passes in a euphoric blur. After the band has played an encore, the lights come on, illuminating beer-sticky floors. I stand in the lineup for the bathroom again. I don't have to go all that badly, but I want to say hi to Sam, thank him for inviting me. It will take him a few minutes to come out. Once again, I squat over the toilet and reapply lip gloss in the blackened mirror. I unwrap a stick of gum and toss the wrapper in the wastebasket. I go back to a table and wait, watching the backstage door. A few minutes later, he swings through it and walks to the bar.

"Hey, stranger," I say, moving in next to him.

"Em, long time," he says, turning and giving me a big hug. He's warm and slightly sweaty from the show. His smell brings back a million abstract memories.

"You guys were amazing, really—wow," I say.

"Thanks, man," he says and grins. "Beer?"

"Yes, please." He orders two from the bartender and hands me a bottle. A few other people approach him to say hi. He turns away. I stand back, holding the sweaty Budweiser and absently picking at the label. I spit my gum into a cocktail napkin and stuff it in my purse. I take a few sips of beer, although I really needn't drink more. Feeling slightly awkward and groupie-like, I pretend to be interested in something on the other side of the bar. The people walk off and Sam turns back to me.

"So, how's LA? I can't believe you live here. Do you have any smokes?"

"I do, actually. LA is good, interesting. I'm adjusting." We turn and walk to the Plexiglas-enclosed smokers' room at the back of the venue. It's disgusting inside. Just breathing in the air is probably the equivalent of sucking back two packs. But you can smoke *and* drink inside here, unlike out in the parking lot. We light up and stand facing each other across a high, round table in the corner.

"So," I say.

"Sew buttons," he says. I smile. He always had a million quirky aphorisms. This one's new to me.

"It's nice to see you, Sam."

"You too, South. Where's that guy of yours? You know I met him last summer at a bar in Halifax."

"Yes, I'm aware."

"He seemed cool. He told me about some crazy porn show he was working on. He still doing that?"

"Yup, he sure is."

"Is that weird for you? Not really your thing, I'd imagine?"

I shake my head no.

"It must be intense to have him be in that world. I wonder what it takes to do that for a living, why people get into it, whether they like it . . . Yeah, lots to think about there." He sips his beer.

Exactly! Yes—a lot to think about! How did Sam nail in two seconds what I've been trying to explain to Robbie for the better part of a year?

"It's kind of all I can think about," I say quietly. We make eye contact and hold it for a minute. His warm brown eyes look calmly into mine. They're kind. A little mischievous. He nods in understanding. "You still seeing the dancer?" I ask.

"Yeah, she's in Stockholm at the moment. Remember that place?" I do remember. He's referring to when we worked as kids' counselors on a cruise ship through northern Europe. It was the summer before we broke up—a rocky time, both figuratively and literally. Stuck in our four-by-four room on E deck out at sea, we fought bitterly. But on our days off, back on land, we were good. We walked Helsinki, Dublin, and Talin together. We both liked Stockholm. We sat in a park and watched all the tall, attractive blondes. We ate extremely expensive Swedish lunchmeat on thick white bread. I smile.

"Things are good with you guys?"

"Long distance is hard," he says. "But yeah, otherwise. Being on the road is tough. You know, everything you hear about touring bands—all the boozing every night and the girls hitting on you?"

"Yeah."

"It's really like that."

"Wow, that must take some restraint."

"All the booze, sheesh." He pats his belly. "I need to watch it. We're getting old, you know. I've been drunk for six months."

"Me too," I say quietly.

"Oh yeah?" he looks at me quizzically.

"Kind of, yeah. Long story." A couple more people enter the smoking room, pushing the crowd closer toward us. Sam slides around the table so that he's next to me now. Our arms brush lightly. We both silently inhale and blow out tandem streams of smoke.

"So you're engaged?" he says.

"I am." I look at him out of the corner of my eye. One summer morning years ago, broken-up but sleeping together again, Sam walked me home to my apartment from his. We were holding hands, shuffling in flip-flops along a Montreal sidewalk, when we made a pact that if both of us still happened to be single in our thirties, we'd make another go of it. Get married. Or just have a kid. It sounded plausible at the time—an insurance plan for our current state of indecisiveness. It was a way to let go but still hold on, just a little—like a toddler dragging around the last shred of a decimated blankey. I liked the idea that everything else in my life could burn up in flames and there would still be someone out there who saw me and knew me. But it doesn't really work like that—the one-foot-in, one-foot-out strategy. Life doesn't wait for anybody.

"How long are you in town?" I say. I want to say: *Let's go walk around the Silver Lake reservoir. Let's go now! We'll sit in the dark and stare at the glassy man-made lagoon until the morning joggers come out, and then we'll laugh at how they're out in Lycra seizing the day's beginning when ours hasn't ended yet. Then we'll go find a taco stand and use our rusty Spanish to order breakfast burritos with Inca cola—remember that diabetes-inducing, electric yellow shit we drank in Ecuador together? What do you say? One last night. One last morning. One last second of incertitude.*

"We're going to spend the day on the beach tomorrow before hitting the road early evening," he says. He butts out his half-smoked cigarette in the overflowing ashtray. "It's pretty nasty in here. Time to get out of the cancer fishbowl," he says. I butt out my cigarette too and we walk back into the bar area.

"Thanks for inviting me," I say.

"No problem," he says. "It's really nice to see you."

We walk together toward the entrance to the club. He turns and looks me in the eyes. We hold focus. Is there something still in there for me? Does it matter? My head swims.

"I should go help them pack up," he says. I nod. He holds his arms out to me. I walk into his hug and breathe him in. He lets go first, smiles a little sadly, or maybe just sympathetically, then turns and walks through the backstage door.

I call Hilary on the cab ride home. My beer buzz is waning, leaving a headache in its wake. "Was I better with Sam?" I say. "Did I get this all wrong?"

"You mean should you be with him? What happened?"

"Absolutely nothing happened, although I can't say I wasn't tempting fate. I don't trust myself right now. Maybe it's not really about Sam—just what he reminds me of. Am I with the wrong type of person? Remember how Sam and I shared a brain, liked the same things, had the exact same sense of humor? You know me, Hil, and you lived with the two of us. Was I a better me with him?"

"Oh, Em," she sighs. Late-night TV is on in the background. I hear the pause before a punch line. Laughter erupts. "Do you want my honest opinion?" she asks.

"Yes."

"Well, you know I liked Sam; we all did. But I think you're better with Robbie. Being *totally* similar isn't always the best thing. Of course you and Sam liked the same movies and music, you dated from eighteen to twenty-three. In a way, we all became who we are as adults together. I think difference helps us grow—but then you're talking a Jew who's dating a Mormon." She pauses; I can hear her exhaling smoke. "Honestly, since you've been with Rob I've never seen you happier. He grounds you."

"Seriously—this is me *happy and grounded*? That's kind of tragic."

"Okay, maybe not this exact second, but in general, yes. Sure, you guys have had your issues, but day to day it just seems so easy. There's a lot of laughter, a lot of love."

"Yeah, I guess there is." I stare out at the passing fast-food joints and strip malls on Hollywood. "I'm sorry to bug you. Thank you. Go back to Tucker. I'll call you tomorrow."

Two days later, I sit in the living room waiting for Robbie to return. My books neatly line the dust-free bookshelf. Since I moved in, they'd collected in piles on my desk or remained half read, abandoned on my cluttered bedside table with lip balm, earrings, and a lamp with a burnt-out bulb. The coffee table is clear, save for a few watermarks that don't come off even with ample Pledge. I did my best. Not a dust bunny lingers. I moved the couch and washed the wood floors underneath. My tornado of clothing is now folded and hung. The kitchen counters, as well as the fridge's vegetable bins, are disinfected. Matt's now-empty room (he'd finally moved into his own place), which I've taken over as my office, is tidy, the blinds dusted and pulled up to invite much-needed sunshine in. I've been busy. I've been scouring for the better part of twenty-four hours, not answering phone calls from Robbie, Kate, or my mom. Not even listening to reggae, my go-to cleaning soundtrack. I have been thinking—tearing up, scrubbing, shaking my head, mumbling to myself, sitting cross-legged on the floor, and then hopping up to mop some more. I burned some sweetgrass my mom gave me to nix any negative, wandering spirits. I have organized my shoes on racks I bought months ago at Target but had yet to set up. I've collected a garbage bag's worth of clothing for the Sally Ann. It's by the door. I even tossed the old cans of Tecate that have lived on the porch for years with the expectation that someone, someday, would return them for money. Not in this lifetime.

I have mostly forgotten to eat, save for a piece of toast with a slice of Swiss cheese late last night, which, for once, has everything to do with anxiety and nothing to do with my wedding dress. Today, it's been nothing but three almonds and an espresso. I have one thought in my head as I wait in the late-afternoon sun for the key to turn in the lock: things need to change. We can't go on like this without collateral damage. I think I've been distancing myself from Robbie in order to feel secure. Some distance is good. But at this distance, we'll wind up leading entirely separate lives with different people. How many days, weeks, or months will I need to ignore him in order to feel okay in my own skin?

Robbie comes through the door with his aviator Ray-Bans on. He's in linen pants, boat shoes, and a pale yellow button-down. "Pass the rum, Panama Jack," I would joke if I didn't have this knot in my throat constricting me. Even dressed like a vacation cliché he looks adorable—sunkissed, skin presumably still salty from one last dip in the ocean before his flight. I want to go to him, take him by the hand to the bedroom, and nap for hours at his side. Forget everything. Couldn't we sort this out with a dose of peaceful silence as we usually do? If only our easy silences hadn't morphed into reckless avoidance over the last eight months.

When Robbie and I were first dating, sometime during the messy bit, he took me up to his mom's country house one weekend. It was fall.

Trees ablaze with bright orange and red leaves enshrouded the cold lake. Lynn and Roger were away; I hadn't met them yet. Robbie's whole world was new to me. Undiscovered. We opened the door to the chilled house, lit a fire, turned on some Neil Young, opened a bottle of red, and began chopping onions and carrots for pasta sauce. I felt giddy and close to him. As usual, we didn't fill the silence with banter. We simply maneuvered in the kitchen side by side, as if we'd always been doing so. At one point, we both put down what we were preparing and turned to each other. Robbie lifted me up by my waist; I wrapped my arms around his neck, hoisted my legs around his middle, and we spun in a dizzying twirl. My view through the glass cupboards became a rainbow blur of mugs and bowls. For a brief second I heard a lucid voice in my head say, *You will marry this man.* I quieted it: *Nonsense, Emily. You just met this guy. Get a grip.* I chalked it up to the wine, the roaring fire, and the bubbling marinara sauce. But I knew I had never felt so elated and yet so calm, all at once.

I stand up from the couch but don't walk to him. I'm afraid that if we touch, I'll collapse and never say any of what I need to.

"Hi," he says, dropping his bag and lifting his shades. "Are you okay?"

"No." He walks toward me. "Can you come sit with me?" I sit on the far side of the L-couch. "We need to talk."

"Okay," he says. He sits on the freshly shampooed cushions of the other arm.

"How was your flight?" I say.

"Fine, smooth. It's really clean in here." He looks around. His blue-grey eyes meet mine with deep concern. "What's up, lovey?"

"I needed to distract myself, so, yeah—no dust mites here! How was the brothel-orgy?" I say, stalling, trying to be lighter than I feel.

"Well, it never happened, actually."

"What?"

"Yeah, they had to cancel it because the strippers didn't have IDs. Then they couldn't find any other last-minute performers. It was weird to go to a strip club and look for girls who wanted to do porn. A lot of them were clearly underage. And they seemed very interested in the money." He shakes his head. "I was really relieved that the shoot never happened."

"You were?" My shoulders drop two inches. My chest surges with relief. Thank God. For once, we seem to be on the same page—the page where we're both not cool with luring teenage strippers into X-rated productions. Maybe this is the resolution I've been looking for. Maybe this revelation makes our situation tolerable. Maybe I can handle just a few more months of this.

"Yeah, not only because of the whole scenario down there; I didn't want to have to come home and tell you about it."

"Oh," I say, suddenly deflating again. So Robbie wants to avoid me as much as I want to distance myself from him. This isn't good. This gulf between us is the real problem—the tangible, negative result his job is having on our relationship.

"It's not easy on me to know that I'm constantly upsetting you." He looks down at his knees and continues, confirming all of my worst fears about where our dynamic is headed: "If I don't tell you what I filmed, which is tempting, then I'm lying to you. But when I do share my experiences, it so often starts a fight. I feel stuck."

"But don't you see? I feel stuck too!" I laugh, but only at the bitter irony.

"What do you mean?"

"Well, if I pretend that the whole culture of porn doesn't bother me, just to avoid discord between us, then I'm losing, because I'm not being true to myself—or to you. But when I'm open about it, it always seems to stir up conflict. Lose again! Sure, I could approach it differently. But I realized something recently. What bothers me most is that we haven't been on the same page. Before you left, when I raised the issue about you going to the Dominican again, you snapped at me that it paid for the ring on my finger. It was like you were throwing my feelings back in my face, and with an intention to hurt. I've been trying to be open about this job for so long, but it's been hard—sometimes impossible. Especially since I've always considered myself very open-minded. I mean, I spent my twenties practicing enthusiastic consent. It's not about sex, Robbie." I chew my lip, forming my thoughts. "The porn industry challenges my values, which is hard to reconcile in this situation. I feel goaded to live up to the ideal these women represent, even if you don't expect me to, and that makes me feel insecure and inadequate. You absorb this world daily through your camera lens. It's like a fucking block of Kryptonite landed in the middle of our living room, and we just keep stepping around it, getting weaker and weaker in its midst, and that terrifies me." I pause, fiddle with my hands, and then look into his eyes and add more quietly, "And then I begin to wonder whether we're even right for each other to begin with."

In that moment, his expression changes. He looks defeated and sad, but worse, he looks disappointed—like I've failed him somehow. It's subtle and fleeting, but real. I have a panicky moment that I've said too much, that I've taken us down a dead-end street instead of the coastal highway of life, and there are no U-turns allowed. *What am I saying?!* But it's out, and I need to hear his answer, because I've put it into the world, this challenge to our compatibility.

Robbie is silent for a protracted minute, taking it all in. Then he takes my hand, his eyes now certain and reassuring. "I love you, Emily, and I want to be with you. I've never been surer of anything." He shakes his head and then continues: "When you say it all like this, I get it. I do. I'm not totally blind to the fact that this has still been bothering you.

I've just felt helpless to change it, so I've compartmentalized it. I put it aside to get through the day."

He goes quiet again. I can tell he's thinking, choosing his words. I stay silent, too, not wanting to rush him. He looks at me out of the corners of his eyes. "Sometimes you *have* seemed okay with this, like over dinner before I left, when we were laughing about Tahitian face masks."

"I know." I give him a half smile, remembering our dynamic that day before it soured. "I have moments when I am. But then something strikes me the wrong way, and I'm back where I started. I don't know how to just say, 'This has nothing to do with me; who cares?' when it's where you go every day. It affects me, it affects us."

He nods. "The funny part is, Emily, I actually appreciate how much you've pushed me to question this world. I'm a lot more aware of the unrealistic standards created by porn and the expectations I've sometimes been guilty of having. I just get defensive when I feel like you're questioning my character. I feel judged. And then my back goes up." He pauses. "But I guess if I'm being totally honest, I do feel a certain pressure to financially support both of us at the moment," he continues, clearly needing to lift a weight off his chest too. "And that's added to the stress of you having a hard time with my job. I've just wanted to put my head down and get through it, just finish out the contract. But I guess putting my head down has actually been exacerbating the situation by making you feel like I don't see what you're going through."

I nod vigorously. He grasps my hand tightly now, so tightly it almost hurts, but I don't want him to let go.

"Are *you* worried I'm not the right guy for you?" he asks. He doesn't let go of my hand, and his eyes glisten with held-back tears.

His question back to me is all the more poignant, because Robbie says—and asks—what he means. It's what I loved so much about him when we met. He was totally straightforward—not sarcastic or obtuse, the way Sam could be. *Funny how we can forget the slings and arrows in the blur of nostalgia.* Robbie wasn't at all like that. He didn't use words he didn't mean or play games. He would always think carefully before he spoke—well, minus the "it pays for that ring" comment. When my mom met him for the first time, she said, "I like this guy. He doesn't let you push him around. That's a first!" She was right; in my own snarky, circuitous way, I was bossy with boyfriends past. My dynamic with Robbie was different. He was direct and said what he needed, as when he broke up with me because I was being wishy-washy and vague. He pushed back. He nudged me out of my comfort zone. We worked, and I loved him.

"I'm positive you're the right guy for me," I say, squeezing his hand back and bumping my knee gently into his. "I like that we're different. I think we complement each other."

"Well, that's good to know," Robbie says, puffing his breath through his lips in exaggerated relief. But we both know this is real, this moment, this test of us. And we both want it to go right, so I push on with what I need to say, even though all I want to do is hold him tight. A wave of nervousness comes over me. It's now or never.

"I want you to quit," I say, as fast as I can spit the words out. "I don't want you to shoot any more porn." There, done. I can't take it back. I stare at the clean coffee table, trace its circular watermark three times around, and then look up. Our eyes meet and now I start tearing up. Everything that's been steeping for months comes streaming down my cheeks in a molten flood.

"Okay," he says calmly. "We're in this together, Emily. You can ask me not to do something."

"I tried to ask you not to go in the first place!" I heave.

"You never came out and said that," he says and brushes a strand of hair away from my teary eyes.

"If I had, you wouldn't have responded well."

"You're right," he says. "I felt like you were being unreasonable because from my perspective it came out as an attack on me, not just the situation. I was being defensive." He shakes his head. "You have to spell things out for me sometimes. But I do know enough to know that we're more important than this stupid job."

"Thanks for saying that," I say. "But, *ugh,* I don't want to have to tell you not to do something!" I say, lifting my hands in the air and flopping them back down on the sofa. "That's the whole point of all of this!"

"But that's not realistic!" he says with equal emphasis. "We're not always going to see things the same way. We can disagree. But you can also veto something, for whatever reason. I can handle that."

"You can?"

"Have you met my mother?"

I laugh. As a teen, Robbie never broke curfew, not once, for fear of his mother's wrath. She's a wee bit intimidating when it comes to protecting her brood—think Anna Wintour meets Florence Nightingale. A force to be reckoned with, but hugely compassionate underneath the chic pants suits. I pull away from him and lean back on the couch. "I don't want to tell you what to do. It's not my style."

"You'd rather insinuate it?"

"Okay: I don't want you to film porn anymore, not right now. There."

"Okay," he says again, nodding his head, firm and certain.

"Just like that?"

"Yeah, just like that. This is you and me, okay?" he says. "From now on we make all decisions together, for real."

I nod.

"Do try not to buy me off with expensive gifts next time," I say teasingly, but also wanting to express how his Valentine's gift came across to me. I wipe my runny nose with my bare arm.

"I really wanted you to have that bike," he says. "Even if it was bad timing."

"I know you did."

"Besides, you may come to appreciate the odd conciliatory diamond in the long run," he jokes.

"I don't want stuff," I say, taking him earnestly. "That's not me. I just want us."

"I know, my love," he says. "I know you."

We're both silent a minute. I can hear a lawnmower whirring outside. A dog barks. He stands and extends a hand. "Come on."

"What?"

"Grab a sweater, let's get out of here."

"Where are we going?"

"I don't know, but do you want to come with me?"

I nod and grab a cardigan from the back of the sofa. Robbie locks up and we walk hand in hand through the bubbling courtyard to the garage.

"Bike or car?" he says, pushing the door opener, which squeaks and grinds as it lifts, letting late-afternoon sun flood in.

"I want to say bike, but we only have one."

"Double you?" he asks.

"Okay," I say. "But you have to go slow."

He raises his eyebrows and rolls up his linen pants above his knees, now looking something like a Cuban Huckleberry Finn.

"Nice look," I say.

"You know you like it."

He pulls Slutty Sue into the back alley and I straddle her cushy, white banana seat. He climbs on in front of me. I wrap my arms around his waist. He balances himself, pushing with one foot along the gravel to gain momentum, and starts to pedal. He turns left at the end of the lane, then right again onto Franklin Avenue. We ride on the sidewalk since we're in LA, after all, where everyone drives, so there aren't any bothersome pedestrians to navigate around. Bougainvillea lines the walls separating homes from the street, which *whooshes* with cars. We cross Franklin, northbound before Vermont Avenue, and cruise through the meandering residential neighborhood. Robbie steers us into the middle of the road. I dig my fingers into his waist. What if a car comes screaming out of nowhere? My legs extend to either side, perilously bare in shorts. Christ, we're not even wearing helmets. Classic us. At least we're no longer twenty five years old and shit-faced—thank God. Nope, we've been through a year of uncommitted dating, two years of long distance, now nearly a year of this. I know we are stronger for it. I dare not tempt fate by saying words like, *forever, everlasting, unbreakable*, but I know now that we have a better shot at this than ever. I bury my face into his warm back and breathe him in—Old Spice, Tide, a dash of lingering ocean water and Hawaiian Tropic. Yeah, a little different, but he's still my guy.

I tilt my head back and relax a little, loosen my grip. Overhead, the sunlit palm leaves flutter against the blue sky. Robbie takes my cue and pumps the pedals faster. We sail alongside lush, manicured gardens and SUVs parked in driveways. He slows and stops as we come up to a red light at Los Feliz Boulevard. Then he turns and kisses me long and hard. Hot and heavy. Just as we did our first night together, years ago. We miss a light, then two. Only breaking apart to laugh when a dude whizzing along in a rusty blue pickup yells, "Get a room!"

After rolling the last few blocks home in the waning sunlight and locking up Sue in the garage, we take heed of the unsolicited advice. We go to our bedroom with no plans to leave it. We close the door, draw the curtains, climb under the sheets, and happily shut out the clamoring world.

AFTERWORD

When Robbie stopped filming *Webdreams*, I sat back and poured myself a tall glass of lemonade—not one of the various booze-inspired concoctions I'd been habitually downing; I suddenly found it easier to relax without three to four doubles. I took a long, deep breath for six months or so. We married in the peaceful chapel at the inn with the blue shutters. We honeymooned in France, where I joyfully reclaimed my love handles scarfing Brie and croissants. We returned to our life in LA. Robbie went off on new, only borderline pornographic projects like *The Hills* and *The Real Housewives of OC*. And I went to work at my job as a Hollywood personal assistant. I took long Sunday rides through Los Feliz on Slutty Sue and began to reflect on what had transpired. I no longer obsessed over my fiancé filming gang bangs. Instead, I calmly contemplated the libidinous acid trip we'd been on; the flashbacks became fewer and farther between, less technicolored. What had happened there? Why had I been so wild-eyed, perched to pelican-dive off the roof over that racket?

If Robbie hadn't worked on *Webdreams,* I don't think I ever would have explored my relationship with porn. Like many, I found the topic too uncomfortable to bring up over cappuccinos and the Sunday paper. Thus, I would have occasionally wondered if he was up in the home office jerking it to *Asian Anal Sluts, 10th Anniversary Bonus Edition,* felt vaguely prickly, and proceeded to avoid talking about it *forever.* Would that have been the end of the world? No. But I'm ultimately glad it didn't happen that way. He is too. (Really, swear on my grandmothers—ask him!) When a couple knows that they don't share the same perspective on a topic—say, politics, religion, or one as potentially heated as pornography—they are probably going to go ahead and steer clear of it. If something turns your stomach, even just a wee bit, you're not likely to suddenly say, "I just love cod liver oil! and start downing the tepid, slippery liquid. Nevertheless, I am proof that forcing the conversation can change your perspective. In the end, the porn show helped me sort out a few of my issues. Who? What, me? *Issues?* Yeah, I guess the feline's already out of the knapsack there.

For starters, I gained confidence in my status in our relationship—sexually and otherwise. I like to know that I'm a priority to my husband. Actually, scratch that, I like to know that I hold the title THE VERY MOST IMPORTANT PERSON IN HIS LIFE. (Have I mentioned that I'm a Leo, like fellow narcissistic lionesses J.Lo and Madonna?)

Anyway, with that established, it turns out I can be an extremely trusting human being of the gentle, compassionate sort. It's when we don't feel secure in a relationship that the crazy comes frolicking over, supremely coked-out in her Stevie Nicks muumuu. It's then that we find ourselves nose-deep in a significant other's email searching for truths, manically Googling a boyfriend's ex-lovers to find out how we compare: *Crap, she was pretty hot. But wait, pear shaped—shaft!* We find ourselves memorizing the layout of attractive females in the room and subtly brandishing the butter knife lest he look the wrong way.

Was Robbie filming porn a real threat to my status as number one? No. Was it a threat to our relationship? Yes. Here's why:

On the one hand, he was merely looking through a lens at some chicks getting busy in their birthday suits, simply capturing their contours in high def. No biggie, right? Except every girl knows that the simple act of a man looking at a woman holds quite a bit of power in our culture. With the whole gender setup the way that it's been for some time now, men have done the lion's share of the looking, and women the better part of getting looked at. (Just as biologically, men do the fucking and women the getting fucked—unless you fancy a strap-on.) A woman knows when she has eyes on her. And she knows when she does not. We gals spend gads of time, money, and energy on captivating the male gaze. *Sure, sure, Oprah, we also primp to be our best selves, and for our girlfriends—the people who actually notice when we get highlights and lose two pounds.* But let's be reasonable: we don't wax, bleach, augment, diet, and wear stilettos *all* for ourselves.

At least I don't. I'd much prefer to laze around with my girlfriends, braiding each other's armpit hair, getting stoned, pounding French fries followed by chocolate-dipped churros, and then magically emerging with a body like Blake Lively's. Instead, I trim, coif, and endeavor to stay svelte. Of course I want men to pay attention to me! And, of course, ideally I'd like my husband to madly desire me *and* find my company scintillating enough not to leave me when my ass resembles an orange peel. I don't realistically think a Brazilian is going to ensure "together forever," but I'd be lying if I said I habitually rip my pubic hair out by the follicles without my hubby in mind. (Note: Robbie read this and called bullshit on the word *habitually.* Thus I feel compelled to admit that I have not currently waxed in nine months. Yup, nine wispy, Woodstock-era months! How about you have the baby next time around, sweetie? Good, then.)

Ironically, the threat back then wasn't Robbie not wanting me because he was comparing me with sexy, uninhibited, naked chicks. Nope, he was perfectly glad admiring *all* of us. The problem was that my sense of self took a beating from all of that *thinking* about Robbie looking at and comparing me with other women. The real threat, in fact, was that I would do something idiotic like firebomb my prospective marriage just to rebalance my perceived loss of power. Chicks—we're so logical! If you had asked me back then, I would have told you that I didn't feel jealous whatsoever. I was a-okay with my guy filming porn. Yup, 120 percent confident. Ha! What a load of hogwilly. I just wasn't sure how to decode the circuitous ways that our situation was affecting me. I didn't know how to communicate my insecurities to Robbie. Turns out "Please stop filming porn because I feel like I want to pull a Lorena Bobbitt!" would have done the trick nicely.

Feeling safe is important. Actually, it's essential in that whole water, food, and shelter kind of way. When we don't feel safe, we are upended. (No, sweetie, I'm not referencing anal sex.) I mean that we are on guard, stuck in fight-or-flight response mode. In retrospect, I can see that that's how I spent the year I was engaged: alternately backing toward the corner with my fists up and keeping the car running, ready to bail. I was defending my place in the world, exerting sexual ownership over my man. Why did I feel the need to do that? Why did I think him filming porn at his day job had anything to do with me?

Something finally clicked while I was listening to Helen Fisher theorize about romantic love on TEDtalks. In her estimation, romantic love is a drive, not an emotion. When we are "in love," changes happen in the brain that are similar to when we have an addiction. Romantic love affects the dopamine center of our brain, the same area triggered by drugs like meth and cocaine. In love, we are high. We can think of nothing else. We obsess over the object of our affections. We earnestly spew platitudes like Bryan Adams: "I would lie for you; I'd die for you." Romantic love is also characterized by extreme sexual possessiveness—a Darwinian impulse to help us lock down a mate long enough to raise children together. *Hmm, that sounds familiar . . .* Alternately, the *sex* drive is more of an itch that begs to be scratched. The sex drive and the kind of deep attachment we have with a long-term mate are both distinctive from the all-consuming force of romantic love. Fisher believes that all three of these things can exist simultaneously and distinctly. We can want to satisfy a sexual urge with someone, be in deep romantic love with someone else, and all the while have a profound attachment to a long-term partner. Surprise, surprise, we're complicated creatures.

To confuse things further, it's easy to conflate sex with romantic love and long-term attachment because of the hormones involved—the spike of dopamine when we are aroused and the surge of oxytocin released when we orgasm. Dopamine, as we all know, feels crazy awesome. And oxytocin, the same yummy hormone women are flooded with in childbirth, encourages us to form bonds of attachment. You can see how one can get confused on this front. In a way, sex does feel like romantic love. Orgasms promote feelings of deep attachment. We can feel an extreme connection to the people we sleep with, if sometimes only very fleetingly. By extension, people can become attached to the feelings they experience via porn. We're also capable of becoming sentimentally involved with donuts, crack, and investment banking. Humans—we're nuts!

In *New York Magazine*'s feature "He's Just Not That Into Anyone," writer Davy Rothbart admits that habitually watching his online gal pals suppressed his desire for the real thing. He felt that some men, himself included, had emotional connections to the girls they were watching on screen. Some preferred getting off to hard-core porn over sleeping with the real women in their lives. At this extreme, porn can certainly be damaging to relationships. Why do you want that fantasyland when you could have the real thing—*me, woohoo, over here?* Nobody wants to hear "The girl on screen does it for me better."

Still, by and large, porn is a consequence-free way to exercise our sexual urges without disturbing romantic love and long-term attachments (as long as you're not a member of any porn-eschewing religion or a hard-core Dr. Phil fan). This makes sense to me now—especially the lifelong attachment part. I think we grow less sexually possessive as a relationship goes on, a glowing ember of sexual jealousy remaining to remind us that our love is not entirely unconditional. Five years ago, I was doped up on romantic love, sexually possessive to the nth degree. It was downright Darwinian of me to want to wrangle Robbie's sexual attention and lock it up kicking in the adobe hut. Except we weren't on the ancient plains, and he wasn't being tempted to impregnate my clanswoman. We were in Los Angeles in 2008. He was filming Internet porn, and I was trying to figure out how to love, marry, and ideally not suffocate him.

A few years later, I can less possessively recognize that my man has various desires. Sometimes said desires are a turn-on, sometimes not, but at the very least, they're not the threat I once perceived them to be. I need not live up to his every whim or fantasy, nor he to mine. I need not run out and max out my credit card on a boob job, some acrylic nails, and a new blonde hairdo at the salon. We've arrived at a place where we can have nonconfrontational conversations about our desires. Much as I was once loathe to admit it, the white-hot attraction of initial romantic love does fade somewhat. *Sigh.* It took me a while not to see this as an automatic negative. I guess that's why they suggest that a marriage is better off if you have some other connections—like playing bridge or a deep abiding passion for couples curling. I'm happy with our sex life these days. Communication and variety help it along. Our run-in with the porn world improved things in this respect. Among other things, I am much more open to recognizing that something that turns me off in one moment can turn me on in another. It means we can check out a squirting (yick, still hate that word!) video together. Have a laugh. Give it a whirl. And not feel bad when I still can't relax enough to master it. *Maybe next year!*

These days, we have a more open dynamic. No topic feels off limits, although I no longer feel compelled to constantly *go there*. Regardless of what we share or don't, our underlying foundation feels more solid. A sexual disclosure doesn't rock the whole boat into the Pacific. For instance, we were sitting by the fire the other day, our three-month-old son gurgling in the bassinet, when Robbie randomly shared a fantasy with me. More, ahem, specifically, he told me he'd envisioned me going down on him and another guy. In his revelry, I then stood up, bent over, and said "Which one of you wants to do me first?"

I appreciated him sharing his daydream with me. It was super-thoughtful of him to make me the girl in the scene, not our neighbor or his coworker. (Seriously, I'm not being glib—it really was considerate. Rule one of sharing fantasies: include your significant other.)

I said: "That sounds fun, sweetie. Maybe we can do that once my perineum heals up from that twenty-one-hour labor."

His fantasy ignited a conversation about power dynamics. He imagined me in control in his daydream. He liked to think that I was the director of the scenario, dictating what was going to happen—when and how, all for my enjoyment. I countered that if this were a porn clip, a hypothetical viewer could easily construe it as male-dominated. There was the sheer numbers game: two dudes, one gal. Then there was the language: "Which one of *you* wants to do *me* first?" Is she catering to them or genuinely asking for what she wants? I know, I know, *Anastasia*, women dig domination. But scenes with women *begging* for multiple members without the foreplay of a private helicopter ride and several glasses of Chablis always strike me as a distinctly male fantasy.

"So should I assume from that statement that every time you want to give me a blowjob, your desire stems from you wanting to fulfill my fantasy rather than from your own desire for me?" my husband asked.

It was a fair point.

"But I never say, 'I want you to ram that thing down my throat till I vomit! More! Deeper! More!'" I countered.

"Feel free to do that," he said. "I won't judge!"

We went around in a circle a few more times. Then we ate some Triscuits with pâté and put the baby to bed. We wouldn't have had this amenable fireside conversation pre–porn show. Could my life have been perfectly swell without this conversation? Sure. But it's moments like this when I feel grateful that I pushed my prudish limits. There was an open field hidden on the far side of the woods. I'm much happier in the clearing.

A few years ago we were two-stepping to a clichéd dance of the sexes. Man wants his privacy around a certain subject; woman heartily prefers to discuss and overthink it to death. Personally, a guy who absolutely would not talk about something like porn with me would be, as they say in advice columns, a deal-breaker. Robbie attests that he's glad he looked into his relationship with XXX. Not because it was a problem before all this happened. But he was carting around a moderate wheelbarrow-load of secrecy and shame about the subject, just as I was hauling around my preconceived notions and judgments. He was worried about how I'd react if he brought something up. It was a self-perpetuating cycle: He felt judged, therefore kept things to himself. I felt something was being held back from me, therefore probed. *What a freaking nightmare.* We were happy to discard that burdensome routine in a heap by the side of the Hollywood 101.

There was another facet to my overthinking porn—the ethics of it all. I'd be cruising along in my day, feeling pretty okay about things, and then, *whaboom,* something would strike me the wrong way, like him coming home from filming twenty guys cum on a girl's face. Immediately I was back to feeling critical, trying to settle the nebulous politics of it all. Can she really feel empowered? Are they trying to suffocate her? Do they hate her? Whose fantasy is this? WHAT DOES IT ALL MEAN? WHY ARE HER PLATFORM SHOES SO UGLY?!!!!

Let me be the first to concede that I often push my sensibilities on porn. I like to make fun of the tacky sets, questionable attire, unattractive men, bloated boob jobs, and glittery makeup in mainstream porn. But there are clearly tons (millions) of folks who are happy with this product just the way it is. People who don't give a rat's ass if Lindsay Blowhan is wearing three-year-old Aldos or Sergio Rossis when she bends over and takes it in the bum. A good number of these consumers are women, chicks who blithely care not whether that manly member is connected to Jorge or Walter or Sven. Porn satisfies a base, sometimes brutal, animal instinct in both men and women. So what is a male versus a female pornographic fantasy? Are they different?

I think we're about to find out. Numerous studies suggest that women are consuming, enjoying, and beginning to create more porn. Women are exploring their sexuality with the same permission and abandonment that men have had for centuries. Access is creating this equanimity (thanks, Internet!). So here's my particular order: I would like to see prettier rooms with hotter men, women au naturel, fewer close-ups of penetration, and hold the cum shots, please. (And, no, a creampie is *not* the only alternative to a cum shot.) I would like to see people who are having a really rocking good time. I like to think I can tell the difference. But can I?

Three years after the show ended, while I was lounging in natty, hot-pink sweatpants, I caught an *Entourage* episode starring porn star Sasha Grey. Curious about her *other* screen life, I pattered over to my desk and Googled her. I instantly came across a particularly zealous blowjob—Sasha gagging on a dude's member, mascara running down her face while she begged for more. I snapped shut the screen like I'd found a cockroach on my keyboard. Pulled my knees up to my chest, wrapped my arms around them, and sat staring at my laptop. Opened it again. Winced. Closed it. Asked myself: *Why does this feel so violent? How does she feel about making this type of porn?* Various YouTube clips later, I had a better idea of her take on it all.

Sasha, to my surprise, seemed to be a self-possessed young woman who was well aware of the male fantasies she played upon. She made no apologies about her choice of trade. She scoffed at the suggestion that she was on drugs. She insisted that she truly enjoys her work. After watching her speak on the *Tyra Banks Show*, I liked her, and disliked domineering Tyra, who infantilized Sasha and was condescending to her. Why did I immediately assume that Sasha was doing something against her will? Yet again, I'd forgotten the key idea: *Fantasy, Emily—make believe, like Mr. Rogers, only different!* I made assumptions based on my own preferences. Okay, I guess *I* don't go for forceful blowjobs. *Or maybe I'd just like a candlelit, filet mignon dinner before I barf it up on some guy's junk.*

When it comes to feminism and porn, I no longer confuse pro-woman porn with who's in control in a scene. A myriad of different power dynamics turn both men and women on. What matters is that everyone is having fun—or at least a passable, consensual day at work. Feminist porn, according to producer Erika Lust, is about what happens behind the scenes. It is porn that is made with respect for humans, both women and men. Porn created in safe working conditions, with proper pay, and hopefully some decent catering around. I believe that the porn industry, like any industry—oil, clothing, mining—should have regulations. However, I've come to realize that policing someone's motivations for becoming an X-rated performer is ultimately disempowering. It takes away a person's agency to conjecture—this young woman or man must be doing this because they are desperate, on drugs, or have been abused as a child.

The intention is to save people from being disempowered. I get it. The sentiment is commendable. Unfortunately, trying to save people from sex work is usually problematic in practice. It's a value judgment to think that someone only works in porn from a misguided impulse or as a last resort. One thing that Robbie filming *Webdreams* taught me is that many performers *do* love their work. If you believe in an individual's right to choose, and I do, we simply have to take them at their word.

This is not to say that I don't think every effort should be made to ensure that work environments are safe and consensual. Age minimums, STD testing, consent forms—I am all for these measures and more. After that, if a woman consensually allows ten, or ten hundred, guys to jizz on her face in order to buy vegetables or go to college, that's totally her prerogative. If a man wants to use his willy to pay the bills instead of driving a bus or becoming a bank teller, well, that's his right. These motivations are personal, not political—the business of the individual, and perhaps his or her friends and family. I will still cringe when I see porn stars who really look like they'd prefer to be shoveling snow or pulling natty hair out of the drain rather than fucking. But instead of getting all high and mighty and worrying about them, I'll cast my vote by turning the it off.

All of that said, I still find depictions of rough sex hard to watch. That gagging, hair-pulling Sasha Grey blowjob scene is just the kind of material that antiporn feminists like Andrea Dworkin and Gail Dines go to town on. They maintain that porn is harmful to women and that images of forceful sex promote real-life violence. If you'd asked me several years ago, I would have been more sympathetic to their cause. I now have a more sex-positive outlook. I no longer think any pornographic act in and of itself is degrading—not spitting, slapping, choking, or cumming on someone's face. Context is everything. Consent is everything. But when you're watching an image on a screen that for all appearances feels unscripted, sometimes that's hard to remember. And if it's hard to remember for prudish adults like me, then it must be difficult for teenagers to ascertain.

I think education is the answer to this conundrum. Do you want your kids talking about hard-core smut as preteens? Because age eleven, according to *New York Magazine*'s Porn Issue, is when most adolescents today start watching it. I don't particularly want tweens watching acrobatic foursomes, but if they're going to find their way behind firewalls, and we all know they will, I think they should be talking about what they see. Personally, I'd like my son to discuss the topic in sex-ed courses designed by forward-thinking educators like Logan Levkoff, author of *Third Base Ain't What It Used to Be*. We need more learning, more discussion, not less.

"Anyone who thinks porn doesn't influence expectations is an idiot," Robbie exclaimed while cooking the other night. He was trying out a new green curry recipe. I was sitting on a stool at the counter drinking a beer. *I'm fond of this arrangement.* I'd just told him that a girl in my twelve-year-old nephew's class had propositioned him. She hadn't asked him to hold hands. She'd asked if he wanted to have anal sex with her. Why ever did she think he'd want that?

"So that's what the kids are doing these days," I joked.

"Yup," he nodded, as he stirred curry paste into a simmering pot of coconut milk and quinoa.

It's to be expected. Of course, watching women scream in ecstasy when they orgasm creates an expectation for such real-life performances. Of course, never ever seeing a strand of pubic hair makes one expect bare cha chas. I looked over at my four-month-old tripping out on the chandelier and drooling madly in his vibrating chair. Don't get me wrong, I'm a long way off from knowing how to talk to my son about Internet porn. *Lord only knows what will be all the rage by the time I get there.* I swigged my beer. I do know that this experience made me better prepared.

Once upon a time, I wanted Robbie and me to be on the same page about everything. Now I realize that was perhaps asking a bit much. We are different. Our brains are different. Our hormones are different. We very often cannot agree on what to make for dinner. Once we've bailed on deciding what to cook and hoofed it to a restaurant, I often determine I prefer the dish he ordered to mine and he offers to switch with me. I am nothing if not changeable. Thanks, estrogen! One day I might be into something in a fantasy way, say, a threesome. But the next day— after having my period arrive unexpectedly in the dentist's chair, then subsequently noshing a mediocre Cajun chicken wrap from Jamba Juice (the only damn thing in the effing strip mall), and accidentally biting my still-frozen tongue trying to stuff my face while driving on the freeway—I might find the suggestion truly and utterly offensive. *Good luck picking the right moments, luv!*

Okay, now here's the part where I quote *Sex and the City*: You know the episode where Aiden moves into Carrie's apartment? She's having a hard time accepting someone else in her space. His boxes and tools and man products are everywhere, and he won't stop accosting her with questions every time she comes through the door. He wants to know where she's been, whom she saw, what she knows. She feels claustrophobic and needs a moment alone. Since there's no space for that in her ten-by-ten apartment, she asks him if he'll not talk to her for a while. He says, "no problem." She closes the curtain between the bedroom and the living room and takes a deep, dramatic Carrie breath. After a minute or two of sitting on her own, she pulls a one-eighty, wants to know what he's doing. She emerges from solitude and gingerly cuddles up on his lap.

The next day, she sits at her desk in short shorts and stilettos or some shit, lights up a smoke, and jots down some version of the epiphany *Sometimes when you get what you need, you don't need it anymore.*

That is exactly how I ended up feeling about Robbie quitting *Webdreams*. After I asked him the thing that was so hard for me to ask, my anxieties lifted. Could putting my foot down to begin with have avoided all these shenanigans? Sure, but then I wouldn't have confronted why I felt uncomfortable about porn, and I wouldn't have the comfort level I now have with my husband.

At times, I wonder if the same job came along again whether I'd be cool with him taking it. About a year ago, Robbie came home one evening from yet another reality TV show he was shooting and said, "Guess what I did today?"

"You bought laundry detergent!" I said. We'd run out a week prior and the lack-of-underwear situation was rather dire.

"Shit . . . No. I shot some porn," he said.

"Oh yeah—where? Why?"

"Our main character was designing a tequila bottle that this porn star Jessie Jane was launching. So we ended up on set with her while she did a lesbian threesome."

"Huh, how was that?" I said.

"Whatever—kind of boring. Are you okay that I did that without asking you? I didn't know that's what we were going to be filming. It all happened fast."

"I'm okay with it," I said. "I'm hungry. What should we eat?"

"Maybe Thai?"

I was ravenous. But wait—was I avoiding my feelings about what he'd just said? I observed my gut to see if there were any cresting waves. The coast was clear. I checked my heart for a small hive of buzzing bees. Nope, not a murmur. That Tuesday evening I really, genuinely didn't care. But then again, the bigger thing I'd learned along the way was that my feelings about porn are not static. On another day, I might feel differently, and so be it. More importantly, I'd come to know what I needed in our relationship to feel safe, respected, and heard. Not safe like, *I will guard the cave and fend off intruders with my manly lance.* Or respected like, *I will never, ever desire anyone but you.* Just heard by a compassionate voice that says, "I know we will see some things differently, but I will try my best to meet you halfway, put you first, and let you in on my life."

Robbie accepted my crazy, and then I didn't feel so goddamned crazy anymore. From there, we were two trees with the wind blowing between us. Suddenly it was all kinds of breezy on Russell Avenue—the palm trees shimmered and swayed. We could begin our married life.

ACKNOWLEDGMENTS

I would like to extend a walloping thanks to my agent, Chris Bucci of Ann McDermid & Associates, for picking up *Prude* and patiently finding it a home. You're the tits, Chris. (The balls?) *Oh dear, here we go again.*

A debt of gratitude goes to Krista Lyons and everyone at Seal Press, most especially my editor, Merrik Bush-Pirkle. Thank you for infusing *Prude* with your wise edits and for your inspiring positivity. I won the editor lottery, hands down.

Thank you, Galafilm, for igniting this book idea by hiring my husband on to *Webdreams*. Yup, who knew I'd thank you all for that? But I do.

I am grateful to my amazing girlfriends, without whom I would be left babbling to myself and drinking alone. Many thanks, Sophia, Sarah, Kim, and Ani. Thank you, Leah, for your astute first edits. And thanks so much, Al, for helping me with the very hardest part of this book: the pitch.

Mammoth appreciation goes to my immediate and extended family for graciously encouraging me to put words to this experience. Thank you also for inadvertently participating as characters. Oh, and apologies for exposing more of myself than you'd perhaps like to know, as well as subjecting you to my profane inner dialogue. Cat's out of the effing bag now.

A mountain of gratitude goes to my incredible mother, Anne, who always answers my million phone calls, is an unflagging cheerleader in the face of rejection, and engendered my first love of books. Thanks, Mom.

And of course, this book would not exist if not for you, my love. Thanks for dreaming big with me, Robbie. Let's never stop doing that. I admire and adore you so.

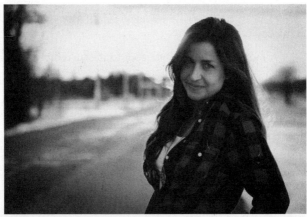

© ROBERT VROOM

AUTHOR BIO

Emily Southwood has written for *The Huffington Post, Betty Confidential, Elle* Canada, and *The Globe and Mail*. She resides in Montreal with her husband, son, and dog. *Prude* is her first book.